State of Health

State of Health

PLEASURE AND POLITICS IN VENEZUELAN
HEALTH CARE UNDER CHÁVEZ

Amy Cooper

UNIVERSITY OF CALIFORNIA PRESS

University of California Press, one of the most distinguished university presses in the United States, enriches lives around the world by advancing scholarship in the humanities, social sciences, and natural sciences. Its activities are supported by the UC Press Foundation and by philanthropic contributions from individuals and institutions. For more information, visit www.ucpress.edu.

University of California Press
Oakland, California

Library of Congress Cataloging-in-Publication Data

Names: Cooper, Amy, 1976- author.
Title: State of health : pleasure and politics in Venezuelan health care under Chávez / Amy Cooper.
Description: Oakland, California : University of California Press, [2019] | Includes bibliographical references and index. |
Identifiers: LCCN 2018037025 (print) | LCCN 2018040640 (ebook) | ISBN 9780520971080 (ebook) | ISBN 9780520299283 (cloth : alk. paper) | ISBN 9780520299290 (pbk. : alk. paper)
Subjects: LCSH: Medical policy—Venezuela—21st century. | Misión Barrio Adentro (Venezuela) | Health care reform—Venezuela—21st century. | Venezuela—Politics and government—1999-
Classification: LCC RC309.P4 (ebook) | LCC RC309.P4 C66 2019 (print) | DDC 362.10987—dc23
LC record available at https://lccn.loc.gov/2018037025

Manufactured in the United States of America

28 27 26 25 24 23 22 21 20 19
10 9 8 7 6 5 4 3 2 1

A version of chapter 2 was published in 2017 as "Moving Medicine Inside the Neighborhood: Health Care and Sociospatial Transformation in Caracas, Venezuela," *Medicine Anthropology Theory* 4 (1): 20–45. A version of chapter 3 was published in 2015 as "The Doctor's Political Body: Doctor-patient Interactions and Sociopolitical Belonging in Venezuelan State Clinics," *American Ethnologist* 42 (3): 459–74.

For Max
Another world is possible

CONTENTS

ACKNOWLEDGMENTS

This book came to life over years of overlapping collaborations with research participants, colleagues in and out of the field, advisers, editors, conference panelists, and friends and family. My deepest thanks go to the Caraqueños who welcomed me into their neighborhoods, homes, and clinics. Their enthusiasm in sharing their stories made this research a pleasure to undertake. In Caracas I enjoyed the support and camaraderie of anthropologists Kay and Franz Scaramelli, Carlos Martinez, Robert Samet, Charles Briggs, and Clara Mantini-Briggs. Charles and Clara oriented me within the health care system and provided crucial contacts on my first visit. Claire Mertz and Katty Aguero proved to be invaluable research assistants, cultural translators, and friends.

Institutional support enabled this research, including fieldwork grants from the U.S. Department of Education Doctoral Dissertation Research Abroad Program, the Tinker Foundation, and the University of Chicago. The Instituto Venezolano de Investigaciones Científicas (IVIC) provided support during fieldwork in Caracas. The Giannino Fund at the University of Chicago, Muhlenberg College, and Saint Louis University funded writing time.

At the University of Chicago Jennifer Cole, Tanya Luhrmann, and Judith Farquhar provided encouragement and influential feedback on project planning, fieldwork, and dissertation write-up. John Lucy, Stephan Palmié, Eugene Raikhel, Jean Comaroff, and Dain Borges also shaped the direction of this research. Staff members Anne Ch'ien, Josh Beck, and Janie Lardner lent crucial support over the years. Fellow graduate students at Chicago provided some of the most useful research insights, including Simon May, Jonathan Rosa, Gustavo Rivera, Lara Braff, Benjamin Smith, Elizabeth Fein, Lily Chumley, Kathryn Goldfarb, Jay Sosa, Aaron Seaman, Julia Kowalski, and John Davy. Participating in the university's Medicine, Body, and Practice workshop and Clinical Ethnography workshop helped sharpen my arguments. As writing group comrades for more than a decade, Pinky Hota and Christine el Ouardani offered comments that greatly improved this work.

At other institutions anthropologists and scholars of Latin America provided feedback and support on this project. Gracious colleagues at Muhlenberg College and Saint Louis University served as sounding boards for nascent ideas. Fernando Coronil, Julie Skurski, and Naomi Schiller helped me better understand the Venezuelan context. Elizabeth Roberts, Raúl Necochea, Kenneth Maes, Janelle Taylor, and Bruce O'Neill each provided insights along the way. Justine Buck Quijada suggested the book's title, *State of Health*. Emily Yates-Doerr shaped the direction of the book with thoughtful comments on the manuscript. Special thanks go to Elise Andaya, who drew my attention to the influx of Cuban doctors to Venezuela in 2003, leading me to change my field site from Havana to Caracas. She also provided invaluable feedback on the manuscript.

Kate Marshall, acquisitions editor, and Bradley Depew, assistant editor, were experts at making each step of the book's production feel both rewarding and stress-free. Kate's enthusiasm buoyed my spirits throughout the writing process and encouraged me to boldly stake my claims. She asked pointed questions where it mattered, forcing me to clarify my argument. Thanks to the artist Manuja Waldia, who created the beautiful cover illustration. Thanks are also due to Sheila Berg for copyediting and Victoria Baker for preparing the index.

Supportive family members in the United States and Ireland (including nonhuman companion, Trotsky the dog) made this project possible. Most important, my husband and the cultural anthropologist, Simon May, made each step of this research immeasurably more successful and enjoyable. In addition to moving to Venezuela for fieldwork and expressing constant encouragement for the project, Simon provided insights throughout the analysis and writing. Nearly every idea in the book was conceived or improved in conversations with him. Thank you, Simon, for all of this and for the life we have together. There really are no words.

ONE

Introduction

MY FIRST EXPOSURE TO VENEZUELAN HEALTH CARE was a dance party in a high school courtyard. Old people grooved to salsa music blaring from a boom box. They passed around pieces of homemade cake and juice spiked with whiskey. Little boys kicked a *fútbol* while the girls took turns riding rusty mountain bikes. They cruised around the rutted concrete, shrieking and skidding to avoid collisions. A contact brought me to the party for my research, but I had no idea why.

I came to Venezuela to study a government health program called Barrio Adentro (Inside the Barrio).[1] Barrio Adentro was a cornerstone of the leftist government of Hugo Chávez that aimed to reverse decades of unequal access to health care by focusing on the poorest and most underserved communities. The ambitious project employed thousands of Cuban doctors to work in neighborhood clinics. As a medical anthropologist I was intrigued by this investment in free and universal access to health care. It flew in the face of global trends in which governments offloaded responsibilities for health care to private companies, nongovernmental organizations, and individuals. No other country was attempting something like Barrio Adentro. This was a historic moment when people experienced a radical transformation in their health care. More than a change in medical institutions, health care under Chávez made disenfranchised people feel valued and empowered by the government. Although Venezuelans' lives have changed dramatically since this period, this book remains a unique account of how poor people experienced this radical social and political change.

This first day of fieldwork demonstrated that studying government health care would mean observing more than what happened inside clinics. At the school that day I met Lilian, a woman with a mane of bleached hair who

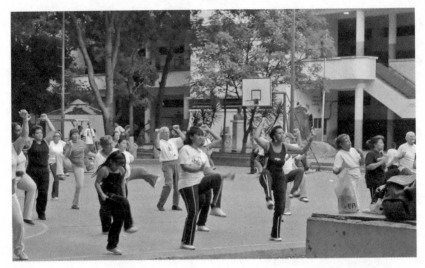

FIGURE 1. Grandparents Club practicing *bailoterapia* in a public school courtyard, 2006. Photo by the author.

presided over the festivities.[2] Lilian's red shirt and cargo vest identified her as a government worker, providing the first clue that what I was observing was not just a party. I explained my desire to research Venezuelan health care, hoping Lilian would inform me about new clinics in the neighborhood. Instead she nodded to confirm I was in the right place, waved her arms around the courtyard, and yelled, "Yes! Yes! Look around, all of this is therapy!"

Only after talking to Darwin, a Cuban sports trainer who welcomed me with a hug and a homemade cocktail, did I learn that the partygoers belonged to a Grandparents Club (Club de Abuelos), a Barrio Adentro program to promote community health. The Venezuelan government employed him to lead dance therapy (*bailoterapia*) classes to help with high blood pressure, heart disease, and other medical concerns (fig. 1). The club was celebrating its members' June birthdays, which explained the refreshments, though subsequent research revealed that *bailoterapia* classes were dependably playful (they just had less cake).

Because people were having so much fun, at first I could not believe this was a government health program. As Darwin led the older adults in a series of vigorous dance moves, some ignored his cues and danced to their own beat. Dancers reached out to people on the sidelines and called out, "¡Baila! ¡Suda!" (Dance! Sweat!). Old women pulled me into their row, demanding that I exercise with them. People laughed and cheered, growing breathless with exertion. When an unexpected downpour began, nobody missed a beat. We hurried up the stairs to a covered stage and continued dancing.

The pleasure that people took in government-sponsored *bailoterapia* classes exceeded the gratification we might expect when feeling our bodies becoming stronger. Grandparents Clubs were fun for their own sake. People took joy in dancing and group outings to the beach. Before Barrio Adentro, they said, nothing like this existed for older adults: a safe public space for socializing and exercising. Some people expressed satisfaction that the government was taking older people's well-being into account after what they perceived as decades of neglect. Knowing that the clubs were government sponsored produced its own kind of pleasure.

When I began research in Venezuela I did not expect to observe people taking pleasure in health care. I definitely did not anticipate writing an entire book about the pleasures of government medicine. Yet as I accumulated field notes and interviews, I was forced to acknowledge that joy, excitement, and satisfaction were central to people's experiences of Barrio Adentro and other government health programs. Participants expressed pleasure even in medical encounters with their doctors, in clinical sites that we typically do not associate with such a feeling.

One example of this is Teresa's story. Teresa was a retired secretary and longtime Santa Teresa resident who experienced encounters with Barrio Adentro doctors as a source of gratification. Teresa seemed proud of her strong constitution and self-reliance, even at the age of eighty-seven. Her petite frame belied an outsized personality that she expressed in impassioned, often belligerent discussions on topics such as the lack of manners among Venezuelan youth and proper fitness regimes for aging adults. Teresa volunteered family remedies for herbal and plant medicine but insisted that she never got sick. She openly scorned pharmaceuticals, saying she did not trust them and did not want their "toxins" inside her body.

Yet by her own admission, Teresa badly needed medical care. She had suffered knee pain for eleven years because she had no money to pay private practice physicians and did not have health insurance through her former employer, where the injury occurred. Teresa also was developing blurred vision. She learned about Barrio Adentro in 2003 from a stranger who noticed her struggling to descend a staircase. At the clinic a Cuban doctor diagnosed her cataracts and referred her for two Venezuelan state-funded trips to Havana for treatment, in which two hundred other Venezuelans participated. The surgeries included airfare, accommodation, and meals for three weeks. Teresa relished her memories of the food, gift bags, and toiletries she received, calling the experience, "Beautiful, totally beautiful!"

A spry yoga aficionado, Teresa was convinced she was right about most things and rarely expressed approval of other people's behavior. She commonly attacked medical professionals she had met in the past for being rude and uncaring. Teresa reserved her rare praise for Barrio Adentro doctors. In field notes recorded after one of my first encounters with Teresa, I wrote:

> "[The Cuban doctors] are very good," she told me. "They will treat you well, spend time with you, and look you in the eyes.... The Venezuelan doctors here are not good. They will never look at you, and they only spend two or three minutes with you." About two years ago she was seeing a doctor, and he was writing down what she said without looking at her, and she confronted him about it.

Teresa explained that doctors in Venezuela often treated poor patients with disdain, but Barrio Adentro doctors (whether Cuban or Venezuelan) treated them with compassion and solidarity. I followed Teresa for a year as her knee was treated in government clinics. She strategized her use of medical sites to get fast and personalized care at each stage of the process. She questioned neighbors and local doctors to find the closest Barrio Adentro diagnostic center that would provide same-day radiology services. After suspecting a hospital doctor of corruption because he told her she had to pay for testing before he could provide a diagnosis, she found another doctor she viewed as more trustworthy at a different government clinic.

A few months after surgery Teresa sought me out and reported she had completed thirty of forty prescribed physical therapy sessions at a Barrio Adentro rehabilitation clinic, demonstrating her progress with some energetic kicks. The eighty-seven-year-old grandmother urged me to acknowledge the intensity and height of her kicks, which she said were all due to the Barrio Adentro doctors. For Teresa, engagements with state medical services were pleasant, vital experiences. She seemed to enjoy the long process of optimizing her body and health. She felt she was receiving the kind of care she deserved.

Teresa understood these experiences of patienthood as politically meaningful. In her memoirs, which she was writing when I met her in 2008, she recorded:

> Thank God! Thanks to President Hugo Chávez, for having consolidated and strengthened Barrio Adentro with all the missions that comprise it. . . .
>
> Doctor Ana Martinez, Orthopedic Surgeon, from the "new generation" of doctors, operated on me, and God grant her long life, energy, and love so that

she can continue working for the poor. She knows how to treat patients with care and respect, and these are the things that every patient needs and yearns for in those critical moments.

Finally, the suffering in my knee has disappeared! ... Do you know how much this kind of surgical intervention costs? From eleven to twelve million bolívares [approx. US$5,200].³ How much did it cost me? Absolutely nothing. They did exams, MRIs, bone density tests, X-rays, electrocardiograms, etc., etc. All for free! I did not spend a single bolívar.

Teresa's astonishment that a government might care about her knee exemplifies a pattern of enthusiasm that my interlocutors expressed about Barrio Adentro. Teresa celebrated access to medical services she could not gain access to in the past. She took pleasure in encounters with government doctors and government medical care that exceeded their therapeutic results. Her memoirs commented on the significance of being taken seriously by the state. Teresa was free from the pain in her knee, but she was also excited because the government was treating her (and people like her—"the poor") as deserving of compassionate medical care.

Health care was a deeply political issue for poor Venezuelans who, like Teresa, had long lacked reliable access to adequate biomedical care. Biomedicine refers to what many in the United States simply call "medicine," which is rooted in biology and physiology. Biomedical professionals like doctors and nurses focus on curing diseases by means of technical interventions. I sometimes use the term "biomedicine" to clarify what I mean because many medical traditions coexist in Venezuela. Teresa and other poor people might not have had access to biomedicine, but they relied on a variety of other healing practices and specialists.⁴

Historically, Venezuelan society was divided along stark class lines. Vast income inequalities meant that while a small elite enjoyed access to high-quality private biomedical clinics whenever they needed them, the majority poor and working classes often suffered long lines, indifferent doctors, and inaccessible treatments from an overstretched network of public hospitals. This dynamic began changing at a moment of significant political upheaval in 1998 when Hugo Chávez won successive national elections by emphasizing the injustice of socioeconomic inequalities and promising to redistribute national wealth. Never before had a radical, pro-poor, leftist president been elected to power. He promised to empower historically disempowered groups—the poor, indigenous people, women, Afro-Venezuelans—exciting people who felt excluded from formal politics. Chávez spoke directly to these people and promised them a greater role in determining their quality of life and the shape of their government. Barrio Adentro was a big part of the government's promised changes, the idea being to revolutionize health care by making biomedicine community based and universally accessible.

Stories like Teresa's provide insight into how people in Venezuela responded to health care during a high point of government investment in health and suggest that the new programs differed in meaningful ways from preexisting medical services. But as stand-alone stories, they do not explain why pleasure, satisfaction, and excitement were common responses to Chávez-era government health programs. Analyzing these stories systematically in cross-cultural and historical context reveals how ordinary people like Teresa experienced periods of momentous political change. These kinds of responses are not commonly reported in research on people's experiences of health care in Latin America.

PLEASURE IN MEDICINE

Decades of research on how people experience government health care in Latin America show that poor and working-class people, particularly women and indigenous people, often experience humiliation, dehumanization, and disrespect when seeking government medical services.[5] This research argues that engaging with state health care reinforces the marginalization of already vulnerable groups in Latin America.[6] In 1990s Venezuela, Charles Briggs, an anthropologist, and Clara Mantini-Briggs, a physician, observed government officials and the media blaming indigenous people for a deadly cholera outbreak that had in fact been caused by failures in the public health system. Briggs and Mantini-Briggs explain that marginalized groups in Venezuela were victims of medical profiling, which they defined as "differences in the distribution of medical services and the way individuals are treated based on their race, class, gender, or sexuality."[7] These Venezuelans were viewed as "unsanitary subjects" unworthy of access to health care.[8] The anthropologist Rebecca Martinez also documented dehumanizing and unequal treatment among poor Venezuelans, this time among women with cervical cancer in a public hospital in the 1990s. Many consultations lasted less than two minutes, and doctors often failed to speak directly to patients. Doctors did not explain upcoming cancer surgeries or even cancer diagnoses because, as they told Martinez, they figured working-class and poor patients possessed a "low cultural level" that made them unable to process the information.[9] These examples from Venezuela reflect a broader trend: a history of medical anthropology research in Latin America that depicts engagement with government health care by poor people as something to be avoided, not embraced.[10] Unequal access to health care and indifferent, even dehumanizing treatment by medical professionals is widespread in the region, and something that my Caraqueño research participants confirmed was true for them in the past.

Rather than take this pattern for granted, we should ask why anthropologists of Latin America rarely describe government health care as pleasurable or empowering.[11] It seems true that as the examples above suggest, government medicine in the region often entails dehumanizing and unpleasant treatment. Experiencing displeasure and disempowerment in medical encounters seems especially likely when patients are women, indigenous, and poor or working class. At the same time, it is possible that people have positive encounters with government medicine that we have not documented as thoroughly. Twenty years ago the anthropologist Judith Farquhar criticized the field of medical anthropology for failing to pay attention to the positive aspects of health care. Her description still characterizes the field on the whole.

> Reading medical anthropology could easily convince one that medicine everywhere is a pretty grim and ghoulish business. Healing technologies of all kinds seem invariably to address suffering and death, and the apparently universal power relation of "doctor and patient" casts the victim of disease as also a victim of social inequality or of structuring cultural models. . . . I take a slightly different tack, . . . to propose that medical practice might at times be a source not just of domination but of empowerment, not just of symptom relief but of significant pleasure.[12]

A tendency to focus on disempowerment in biomedical encounters reflects a broader trend in cultural anthropology of studying suffering, oppression, and inequality. In 2016 the anthropologist Sherry Ortner declared that the main trend in anthropological research since the 1980s was "dark anthropology," which she defines as "anthropology focused on the harsh dimensions of social life (power, domination, inequality, and oppression) as well as on the subjective experience of these dimensions in the form of depression and hopelessness."[13] Anthropologists have focused on the negative aspects of social life but not because we are all gloomy pessimists. Rather, we have tried to describe the global reality of economic precarity and rising inequalities that seem to increasingly threaten people's ways of life. This research is important because it demonstrates that in spite of cultural differences, people around the world struggle with systemic forms of economic exploitation and oppression.[14]

At the same time, to understand the world in which we live we need detailed research on pleasure, the good life, well-being, happiness, resistance, and empowerment—especially in contexts of historical disempowerment. Focusing on positive as well as negative responses to medical care, for example, can clarify the effects of health policies and government regimes that claim to improve people's lives. Though uncommon, ethnographies that address the pleasurable aspects of health care explore a wide range of experiences, suggesting that pleasure in medicine is widespread and more meaningful than previously assumed. For example, in analyzing the pleasures of recreational and prescription drug use, Kane Race questions the way a moral injunction against taking drugs for pleasure supports an artificial boundary between licit and illicit drug use (we only have to think about Viagra to see the absurdity of strict divisions between recreational and therapeutic drugs).[15] Some scholars discuss the ambivalent status of medications such as Ritalin and Adderall that produce feelings of pleasure in the body while treating a therapeutic need.[16] Others have examined how medicalized spas and medical tourism blur culturally constructed boundaries between "healing" and "holiday."[17] This research shows that medicine and pleasure are connected in spite of cultural assumptions that they cannot—or should not—coexist. In such cases, therapies that clearly elicit pleasure for users might come under attack or gain an ambiguous standing. In other cases, anthropologists have documented how reproductive technologies, specifically, fetal ultrasounds, can be fun and exciting for parents who delight in seeing their baby and anticipate sharing the scan with others.[18] Farquhar has written about how "eating" traditional Chinese medicine serves as a source of pleasure in its own right.[19] Farquhar and Qicheng Zhang examined how Chinese health promotion practices known as the "life cultivation arts" provide social and political satisfaction for elderly Beijingers who can no longer look to the state for health care.[20] Other ethnographic works documenting pleasure in medicine include studies of compassionate interactions with nutrition consultants in Guatemala and private practice IVF doctors in Ecuador, as well as community health workers attempting mosquito control in Nicaragua.[21] If we were to consider healing arts such as yoga and rituals such as ayahuasca ceremonies, we would see more evidence of people taking pleasure in health seeking.

I propose making pleasure an explicit focus of analysis in medical anthropology. Many forms of medicine elicit pleasure, and documenting these would help us understand how people experience medicine in affective terms. We do not know what we will learn by theorizing about the pleasurable aspects of medicine. Using ethnography to explore what brings people pleasure, we may attain a better understanding of how culture and history shape desires for certain material goods, relationships, and experiences. We may be better able to offer comparative accounts of how people imagine and strive to achieve well-being according to distinct cultural logics. My research found that certain political moments give medicine an outsized significance in society, and studying people's experiences of medicine in these contexts provides unique insights into how people experience radical social change more broadly.

Specifically, I propose focusing on pleasure beyond the positive feelings associated with health care's therapeutic effects. We have all experienced pleasure when a treatment worked as promised: when headache tablets provide relief, surgeries improve bodily function, or physical therapy restores mobility. We are pleased when a doctor resolves problems that trouble us or when a medical encounter boosts our sense of well-being. But medicine also produces positive effects unrelated to the therapy received. We could call these feelings the "surplus effects" of treatment.[22] Medicine can evoke a sense of social support, care, and compassion, activate a sense of class mobility, and mark historical improvements in quality of life. In Venezuela under Chávez, government health care affirmed poor people as valued members of society by making it clear that their lives mattered.

Paying more attention to the positive aspects of medicine can revolutionize our understanding of how health care gives meaning to people's lives. In this book I take seriously poor and working-class people's narratives about government health care as a source of pleasure and satisfaction. Many of my interlocutors were not only members of historically marginalized communities, but agents who were actively engaged in forging better lives for themselves. Unraveling the reasons medicine served as a source of pleasure for certain Venezuelans at a particular point in history, this book shows that government health care addressed political and social inequalities by making people feel valued. Theorizing pleasure in this context revealed that people appreciated government medicine as a therapeutic tool and as a technology of social justice.

Defining Pleasure

I use the term "pleasure" because it describes people's experiences of government health care better than terms like "happiness" or "well-being."[23] All of these concepts refer to experiences or states of being that are deeply dependent on cultural meanings: what produces pleasure, what counts as happiness, and how people assess well-being vary across cultures and historical time. Yet while happiness and well-being reflect states of being based on a holistic assessment of one's life, pleasure typically describes responses to discrete, time-limited experiences such as eating a meal, having sex, enjoying an artistic performance, taking a mood-altering drug, or undergoing a religious ritual. And while happiness, well-being, and pleasure all develop in relation to external circumstances, only pleasure refers specifically to an embodied experience of the material world. In this book I focus on the types of pleasure people take in tangible embodied activities related to government health care, things like dancing in a public plaza, hearing a kind word from a government doctor, and filing paperwork to help a neighbor obtain a medical device. These kinds of activities elicited pleasure from participants that was culturally and historically meaningful.

We can observe people enjoying medical encounters in a number of health care settings globally—likely for a variety of reasons—but pleasure in the Barrio Adentro program pointed to important and specific meanings. Venezuelan government health care elicited pleasure among poor and working-class Venezuelans for three distinct reasons. First, increased access to medical services produced material improvements in their biophysical health. This was the most straightforward and expected outcome I observed. Of the hundreds of patients I met, the vast majority volunteered reports of improved physical health that they attributed to expanded government health care. Pragmatically this is what we hope for from health reform: better access to care and improved health as a result. Alongside expressions of pleasure about improved access to medicine, however, I also observed complaints that reforms were incomplete and inconsistent. The same people who praised the new system often called for it to expand and improve. That people hoped for and aspired to even more government health care does not negate the material impact of Barrio Adentro or the positive response it elicited.

Second, government health care produced sensual and social pleasures. Examples of sensual pleasure include treatments that improved one's bodily experience of the world. Patients described caring government doctors who, unlike doctors they had encountered before, looked them in the eyes, joked and used pet names with them, and offered compassionate touches or hugs. For many, this kind of care held sensorial and social meaning; patients seemed to cherish doctors who practiced personalized, intimate clinical interactions. Grandparents Club members took pleasure in the exertion, sweating, socializing, and fun of dance therapy classes and field trips. People who became community health workers in Barrio Adentro displayed high spirits when collaborating on a door-to-door census or developing friendships with each other in a government training session. Participating in government health care had positively valued effects on the body and sociality that exceeded the biophysical improvements brought about by medical services. These effects seemed to be valued for their own sake.

The third source of pleasure was political. Patients and health activists expected health programs to do more than cure disease: they saw participation as a means to sociopolitical empowerment. In spite of their problems, government health projects elicited excitement and pleasure because they identified marginalized Venezuelans as bodies that mattered. This finding forms the heart of this book. While any Venezuelan might enjoy experiences of improved biophysical health or the sensual and social pleasures of exercise, only the disenfranchised found government medicine politically empowering. This book aims to explain the meanings of medicine from the vantage point of historically disempowered Venezuelans in particular—poor people, people of color, and women, among others. These groups make up the vast majority of Venezuela's population, which is why this story is so important. If we want to understand how ordinary Venezuelans experienced the Chávez government during this period, we should look at their experiences of Chávez-era health care.

Historically, only certain social groups enjoyed dependable access to biomedical care in Venezuela. Because social inequalities mapped onto unequal access to health care, access to decent biomedicine was associated with wealth, power, privilege, and participation in the formal economy (the latter because only certain kinds of work allowed access to Social Security medical services). My interlocutors took pleasure in the fact that "people like them" (i.e., members of the poor and working classes) could enjoy more reliable access to medical care through Barrio Adentro. Improved access to health care marked increasing social equality. This fact pleased and gratified people from marginalized backgrounds.

Prioritizing community health also meant establishing government clinics in marginalized neighborhoods, which helped resignify those neighborhoods in positively valued ways. Patients felt that clinics identified historically stig-matized barrios and the people living there as worthy of the state's care while publicly resignifying neighborhoods as capable of promoting health rather than endangering lives through violent crime and lack of services.

Tens of thousands (possibly hundreds of thousands) of Venezuelans par-ticipated in community health work for the Barrio Adentro mission. Participation offered volunteers opportunities to help other people and revi-talize their communities, both highly valued forms of activism. Being a health promoter evoked pleasure and feelings of satisfaction among people who felt they were heeding the Chávez government's call to play a role in revolutionary democratic political processes. This was the pleasure of belong-ing to a movement bigger than oneself, being caught up in a revolutionary moment symbolic of broad social changes.

For nearly a century, the Venezuelan state had presented itself as a "magi-cal state"[24] that redistributed the nation's oil wealth in the form of develop-ment projects for the benefit of all citizens. Political leaders framed citizen-ship as the shared ownership of oil wealth and cultivated expectations for a wealthy state that would provide for its people. Yet for most poor people and particularly during the 1980s and 1990s, when neoliberal policies were in place, the government failed to live up to its promises. During the heyday of Chávez-era government spending when Barrio Adentro was rapidly expand-ing, patients felt their concerns were being taken into account not just by medical professionals, but by the state itself, interrupting a history of margin-alization with practices that reflected inclusion and belonging.[25]

Culture and history shape many of the pleasures I identify. A Venezuelan mother might express a strong sense of gratification at receiving free medica-tion for her children due to a history of past deprivations, while somebody who has had access to free health care her entire life might not feel or express gratification for the same benefit. Expressions of pleasure in government health care also reflected the broader political climate of Venezuela at the time. The country was politically divided between people who saw value in Chávez's vision of socialism, which meant empowering the historically dis-enfranchised majority, and people who did not see value in this vision. People who expressed pleasure in specific aspects of government health programs were often expressing their approval of the government itself (the reverse was often true). If you learned how to read them, expressions of pleasure in health care communicated claims about the rights of citizenship and gratification at being taken into account.

Analyzing why people found health care a source of pleasure challenges reductionistic analyses that assume health care's sole purpose is to address biophysical health concerns. In the case of Barrio Adentro, expressions of pleasure serve as a key to understanding broader cultural, social, and political desires and aspirations among a majority of Venezuelans. Certain aspects of health care beyond medicine prompted pleasure and activated a sense of political belonging. With Barrio Adentro, the location of clinics, how doctors behaved, the freedom to integrate new health programs into existing practices, and participating in community revitalization all produced a meaningful experience of social and political change.

OIL AND EXPECTATIONS IN VENEZUELA

In order to understand why the Barrio Adentro program was pleasurable and politically significant we must understand Venezuela's history, especially how oil wealth shaped people's expectations of their government. A long-standing promise by state officials to share the nation's oil wealth established the notion of a Venezuelan birthright that persisted throughout the twentieth century in spite of numerous government failures to use that wealth for the benefit of the people. While enthusiasm for Barrio Adentro reflected a historical hunger for health care, it also reflected a long history of expecting and desiring state services funded by oil wealth that was perceived as the rightful inheritance of all Venezuelans.

Expectations of Citizenship

Venezuela possesses the largest oil reserves in the world, with nearly 300 billion barrels of proven reserves. It would be hard to overstate the impact of this vast source of wealth on economic, political, and social relations over the past hundred years.[26] Politically, oil defined Venezuelan society by allowing successive generations of politicians to promote a model of citizenship in which national belonging meant enjoying a share of the nation's wealth.[27]

Starting in the 1930s, politicians framed state investment in infrastructure, agriculture, and other economic and social projects as distributing the country's oil wealth to the people. They coined the phrase "sowing the oil" (*sembrando el petróleo*), denoting a political commitment by the state to extract the nation's wealth and distribute it to the population by means of economic and social development projects. These distinctively Venezuelan ideas of citizenship shaped what people came to expect from the government.

For almost fifty years the Venezuelan state rolled out economic and social development projects bankrolled by oil profits. State interventions to promote social welfare during this period included price controls for basic goods, minimum wage laws, and subsidies for gasoline, public transportation, and utilities. In the field of health care, "sowing the oil" entailed national immunization campaigns and expanding the public hospital system and local medical centers. These initiatives led to notable gains in people's quality of life, measurable as a steadily falling infant mortality rate, a higher life expectancy, and the eradication of diseases.[28] With oil profits flowing, Venezuela enjoyed the highest per capita income in Latin America. This marked wealth, in addition to an uninterrupted period of democratic rule from 1958 on, led many scholars to argue for what became known as "Venezuelan exceptionalism" in Latin America.[29] Encouraged by state promises and government interventions, many Venezuelans felt entitled to continued improvements in their living conditions.

Persistent Inequalities

Dazzling wealth and narratives of progress helped hide the fact that people did not share equally in the nation's prosperity. When the global oil market soared, oil windfalls enabled government spending bonanzas like one in the mid-1970s that alluringly promised to deliver "the Great Venezuela." But in spite of impressive assets and ambitious development projects, Venezuelans suffered one of the worst levels of income inequality in Latin America.[30] This unhappy status quo persisted for decades while entrenched political parties suppressed grassroots and leftist organizations that sought a role in political decision making.[31] Meanwhile, state interventions never established a comprehensive social welfare system.[32] Social programs were circumscribed and unevenly distributed. Health care offers a good example of this problem. Venezuelans faced a byzantine, fragmented system of public and private health care. In 1973, over one hundred government institutions provided public health care, with the main players being the Ministry of Health (MSAS), the Social Security Administration (IVSS), the military (la Sanidad Militar), and the Ministry of Education.[33] Poor and working-class Venezuelans relied on the government for biomedical care, but many people fell through the cracks of the fragmented system.

A 1983 study of a government-run clinic reveals the limitations of poor people's access to biomedicine.[34] Located in the barrio of Petare in eastern Caracas, El Libertador health center was part of an initiative to bring public services to barrio residents during a period of heightened state spending in the 1970s. The doctors were recent graduates of the Universidad Central de Venezuela assigned to complete their obligatory year of service work (physician turnover rates were high). Patients praised the doctors for their earnest and thorough medical exams in spite of the fact that their prestigious medical training did not prepare them to provide basic services in high demand among barrio residents, like family planning. The center hired a psychologist, a social worker, and a dentist and organized weekly doctors' visits to remote parts of the barrio. Yet major problems plagued the clinic. Administrative failures to deliver supplies meant well-woman exams were cancelled for five months in 1983. The jeeps used for doctors' visits broke down and repair requests went unanswered. Doctors' attempts to help patients receive diagnostic tests and treatments at other public facilities often failed. The clinic was built on the edge of its catchment area, making access difficult for at least half its population. Zoned for an area with 20,000 residents, the clinic had only 3,000 registered patients after more than a year in operation, meaning only 15 percent of barrio residents used it.

Social inequalities and poor people's access to services like health care got even worse when oil prices fell. A series of interconnected economic crises unfolded in the 1980s and 1990s; inflation, government corruption scandals, a banking crisis, and massive amounts of capital flight crippled the economy. External debts that the government accumulated during the 1970s oil boom soared to give Venezuela the highest per capita debt in Latin America.[35]

During this period the country came under foreign pressure to adopt neoliberal austerity measures. Neoliberal ideology assumes the efficiency of free market thinking across a range of human activity and advocates dismantling state welfare systems to make social welfare the responsibility of individuals and private industry.[36] Now hegemonic in many parts of the world, including the United States, neoliberalism promotes a model of state and society that undermines the Venezuelan model of state-led intervention for social development.

Venezuelans rejected a model of economic development that denied that national wealth was the people's birthright. In 1989 voters elected a president who explicitly campaigned on an anti-neoliberal platform. Yet he quickly reneged on his promises and accepted an International Monetary Fund

(IMF) loan in exchange for implementing government austerity measures that ended subsidies for things like gasoline and public transportation. The day after the IMF agreement was announced, massive looting and protests broke out across the country, especially in Caracas. State security violently repressed protesters, most of whom were poor, and buried many of its hundreds of victims in a mass grave.[37] The event came to be known as the Caracazo and was a turning point in Venezuelan history, marking people's loss of faith in conventional democratic processes to resolve social inequalities.

In the years that followed, the myth that Venezuela's national wealth would promote social progress broke down as economic crises and neoliberal reforms led to a dismantlement of state welfare programs. The government cut public spending, reduced price controls and subsidies, and implemented policies that led to restricted wages and precarious employment.[38] Venezuela suffered under neoliberalism much as other Latin American countries that experimented with these policies. Venezuelans saw their standard of living fall dramatically across the 1980s and 1990s. Between 1984 and 1991, poverty rates nearly doubled, from 36 percent to 68 percent.[39] In the field of health care government spending fell dramatically with an expectable deterioration in health services.[40] The state began dismantling national health services by decentralizing them, forcing states and local governments to charge fees for health services due to lack of funding.

Neoliberal policies restricted access to health care during a period of prolonged economic crisis—just when people needed it most. Diseases believed to be eradicated reappeared, and infant mortality rates, which had been dropping steadily in previous decades, started to rise.[41] A 1998 national survey found that 80 percent of people with chronic health problems could not afford their medications. As in other countries that implemented neoliberal reforms, social inequalities became more marked. In Caracas, infant mortality in the poor municipality of Sucre was six times higher than in the adjacent middle-class municipality of Chacao.[42] Poor and working-class areas grew more socially and spatially segregated from middle-class and wealthy areas in Caracas as fears of crime and a generalized fear of the poor (tied to memories of looting during the Caracazo) led people in wealthier neighborhoods to install exclusionary security measures like walls and guard stations.[43]

Neoliberal policies were extremely unpopular among Venezuelans. People lost faith in a political system that they now viewed as inefficient, corrupt, and unresponsive to their needs and expectations. A poll taken in 1998 found that "more than 85% of Venezuelans felt cheated out of the benefits of oil wealth."[44] The Caracazo, the largest popular protest against neoliberalism in Latin America, heralded the beginning of a decade in which Venezuelan voter abstention was high and "street politics" (*la política de la calle*) dominated as a means of expressing political demands.[45] Between 1989 (the year of the Caracazo) and 1999 (the year Hugo Chávez became president), students, senior citizens, housewives, medical professionals, street vendors and others staged over seven thousand public protests.[46]

When a political outsider and young military officer named Hugo Chávez led a failed coup attempt in 1992, his critiques of social inequality and promises to end government austerity captured the public imagination. After serving time in prison, he entered formal Venezuelan politics, winning the presidency by a double-digit margin in 1998. Barrio Adentro became one of the largest and most important of his social welfare programs, framed as a state intervention to use oil wealth to improve people's lives and promote social justice. By funding Barrio Adentro and other social programs with profits from the national oil company PDVSA, and improving people's quality of life, people felt the government began to actualize the promise implicit in its new motto, Venezuela: Ahora es de todos (Now Venezuela belongs to everyone).

The Promise of Change

With approval ratings of up to 90 percent at the time he took office, Chávez enjoyed an obvious mandate for the systemic changes he promised.[47] His first major act was to organize a constitutional assembly to transform the legal and philosophical underpinnings of the nation-state. People nationwide elected the constituent assembly and engaged in organized public debates, directly participating in constructing the new constitution.[48] Venezuelans approved the new document by 72 percent in a popular vote. The 1999 Constitution was socially and politically progressive, emphasizing direct political participation for historically dispossessed social groups, including women, Afro-Venezuelans, and indigenous peoples. The Constitution provided universal guarantees of access to health care, housing, employment, and education (fig. 2). Chávez coined the term "Bolivarian Revolution" (after the liberator of Latin America, Simón Bolívar) to describe the dramatic social changes he sought to implement.

Talk of a revolutionary Venezuela alienated some people, especially members of entrenched elite groups.[49] Political animosities grew intense and uncivil. In mainstream newspapers and television shows, opposition to

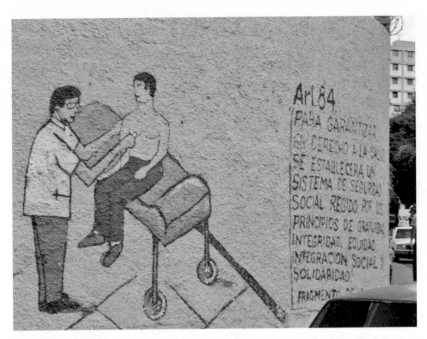

FIGURE 2. Mural of a doctor's visit alongside Article 84 of the 1999 Constitution guaranteeing state-provided health care, 2006. Photo by the author.

Chávez devolved into racist attacks comparing him to a monkey because of his Afro-Venezuelan and indigenous heritage.[50] Chávez and his supporters derided their most fervent opponents as *escuálidos,* "squalid ones." The right-wing opposition repeatedly tried to oust him from office via legal and extralegal means. Their efforts included a failed coup attempt in 2002, an oil industry strike in 2003, and a recall referendum in 2004. In facing down these challenges, the government gained more supporters. Chávez won reelection in 2006 with 63 percent of the vote, with a 26 percentage point margin of victory and twice as many votes cast for him compared to 1998.[51]

Resisting destabilization and gaining confidence from his reelection, Chávez radicalized his politics. He discussed the country's transformation from capitalism to what he called "twenty-first-century socialism." He strengthened ties with Cuba and established trade and aid programs to benefit countries in Latin America and the Caribbean. A few years earlier, the government had founded a string of national social programs called *misiones socialies* (social missions) to fulfill constitutional guarantees to health care

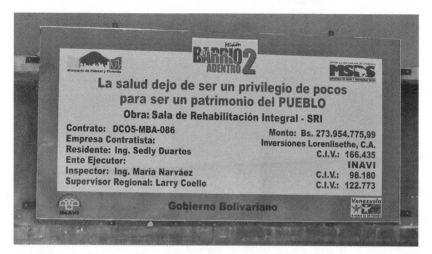

FIGURE 3. Construction site for a Barrio Adentro rehabilitation clinic, 2006. The sign reads, "Health is no longer a privilege of the few—it is now the patrimony of the PEOPLE." Photo by the author.

access, education, and other benefits (fig. 3). Using the language of missions marked them as distinct from other government social programs. The term "missions" invoked Catholic and evangelical Protestant mission work and the concept of a revolutionary mission that imbued government welfare with moral connotations of compassion and social justice. The missions received direct funding from PDVSA, activating long-standing promises to "sow the oil" for the benefit of the people. Between 1998 and 2006 government social spending increased by over 200 percent as officials rolled out new programs across the country.[52] Using oil profits to fund social programs also reflected a commitment to repay the "social debt" owed to people after the ravages of government austerity. Unlike the idea of "sowing the oil," the concept of social debt is not unique to Venezuela. Across much of Latin America the idea gained traction as a way to highlight states' obligation to redress social inequalities that their neoliberal policies inflicted.[53]

Barrio Adentro

The centerpiece of the Bolivarian Revolution's efforts to address inequalities and repay the social debt was Barrio Adentro. The Barrio Adentro mission provided universal primary and preventive health care with a focus on under-served communities. As of 2014, this Venezuelan and Cuban government initiative had approximately thirty thousand Cubans working in Venezuelan clinics and training Venezuelan medical students (most of whom came from poor and working-class backgrounds) to practice community medicine.[54] Barrio Adentro began as a pilot project in the Libertador Municipality in 2003 when the municipal mayor invited Cuba to send doctors to staff the new program after recruitment of Venezuelan doctors failed (presumably because they were disinterested in working in poor neighborhoods far from home).

While turning to a foreign government for medical workers might seem odd, it made sense in this context. Cuba enjoys a well-earned reputation for medical internationalism, having sent doctors to live and work abroad for over fifty years. Just a few years before, 450 Cuban medical workers provided relief aid in a coastal zone near Caracas after a natural disaster killed and displaced thousands of residents.[55] Revolutionary Cuba has consistently prioritized population health at home, producing an extensive community-based medical system, a high doctor-patient ratio, strong infant and maternal health indicators, and continuous health education campaigns. Cuban medicine is rooted in claims that health care is a basic human right and that improving people's health promotes equality and social justice. These beliefs formed the moral basis of Barrio Adentro as well.

Borrowing from Cuba's community-based Family Doctor program, Barrio Adentro established approximately six thousand primary care clinics across Venezuela.[56] It included three levels of health care. Neighborhood primary care clinics (Barrio Adentro I) provided free basic health care, immunizations, well-woman care, referrals for testing and specialized treatment, and approximately one hundred different medications. The model called for a single doctor and nurse to staff each clinic. Dentists also worked in some Barrio Adentro I clinics. Specialized health centers (Barrio Adentro II, CDI and SRI) offered diagnostic and rehabilitation services at no cost: X-rays, mammograms, blood and other lab work, MRIs, and physical therapy, speech therapy, acupuncture and other forms of physical rehabilitation. The third level (Barrio Adentro III) was intended to rehabilitate and expand the government hospital system but was the least developed of the three.

Nearly all my research participants praised the idea of Barrio Adentro because it resonated with religious, political, and medical discourses in the region about who should be able to access biomedicine. Regionally, a shared conviction that health care should be available to all regardless of ability to pay is informed by Catholic notions of healing, charity, and vocational work; liberation theology; the influence of politically progressive scientists and doctors; and a history of leftist and populist programs to implement national health care.[57] Venezuelans across socioeconomic classes favored the idea of universal public health care, and contemporary political candidates, even those hostile to the revolutionary government, debated how the state could ensure universal access, not whether it should do so. A recent survey of barrio residents found that they viewed state-guaranteed access to health care as one of the most important features of the country's democracy.[58]

Yet Barrio Adentro stoked immense political controversy. The mission's use of Cuban workers, its administrative status outside the Ministry of Health, and its political identity as a "Chávez project" drew critics, especially from the Venezuelan medical establishment.[59] Cuban doctors, who made up 80 percent of doctors working in the program, faced accusations that they were not properly certified, not well trained, or not doctors at all but communist infiltrators.[60] Another common complaint was that funds used for Barrio Adentro siphoned money from other government health services. These critiques dominated global media reporting on Barrio Adentro, framing the program as poorly conceived and crippled by its own failures. Domestic opposition to Barrio Adentro dissipated as it gained widespread popularity, but its political significance made it a target of scapegoating during times of national unrest, when isolated cases of verbal and physical assaults on Cuban doctors and attacks on Barrio Adentro clinics (including vandalism and arson) occurred.[61] This dynamic continues to the present day, with violent attacks on government clinics and hospitals forming part of wider protests against the socialist government of Chávez's successor, Nicolás Maduro.

The Present Day

Chávez maintained popular support for his vision of a more equitable Venezuela, remaining president until he died of cancer in 2013 at the age of fifty-eight. The current leader, Maduro, ostensibly would follow in Chávez's footsteps, though in many people's view Maduro failed to live up to expectations for a revolutionary government that improves the lives of the disenfranchised. Facing more widespread criticism for his leadership style and decision making, Maduro has yet to successfully address the ongoing economic crisis that began around the time he took office and contributed to violent protests by the conservative opposition and a significant decline in people's quality of life.

In the wake of recent crisis, social programs faltered in their promises to uplift the poor. Health care improvements from the Chávez era have come under threat. Everyday experiences of health and life deteriorated in the shadow of economic despair. The book's conclusion offers a more detailed analysis of the present day. I acknowledge these changes here because one should understand that the high-spirited engagements with health care that this book documents belonged to a political moment that has passed. This story remains crucial, however, because it reveals how people experience radical social upheaval and political change. One of the unique aspects of this research is its analysis of how feeling valued by state institutions can transform people's sense of themselves.

Measuring Health and Well-Being

This is not a book about whether or not the Barrio Adentro program was successful. Nor is it a book about whether or not Barrio Adentro improved health outcomes and lives. Rather, it is a book about how individuals experienced health care as a mechanism of social inclusion and empowerment. In other words, this book explores the extramedical meanings of government medicine.

At its core, this book answers the question, why were Venezuelans so happy to go to Barrio Adentro doctors? But one of the most common questions people ask me about Venezuelan government health care is simply, did it work? While the former question interrogates what health care means, the latter question asks what health care does, such as whether Barrio Adentro improved access to health care or whether it improved population health. Some readers believe that what a health program means is less important than what a health program does, and whether it is sustainable.

Although the intent of this book is not to evaluate the success of a health care project, I can provide some context for those who want to know if it worked. Undoubtedly, the mission improved access to health care. My informants consistently reported this, and their claims were borne out by national data. The year before Chávez was elected president (1997), private spending on health care made up nearly three-fourths of all health spending in Venezuela. After Chávez took office, between 1998 and 2007, the number of government primary care clinics in Venezuela tripled.[62] Nearly all of them were built in areas that had minimal or no government health presence before. Between 2004 and 2005 alone, Barrio Adentro reportedly provided 150 million medical consultations.[63] The doctor-to-patient ratio increased from 20:100,000 to 80:100,000 between 1999 and 2014.[64] Three years after instituting Barrio Adentro, the program was providing health care to 17 million Venezuelans (63 percent of the population), while the preexisting government medical system provided care to another 3.5 million people (13 percent of the population).[65]

Assessing whether Barrio Adentro has improved population health is a difficult undertaking. Measuring health and attributing changes in health to specific interventions are challenging. Medical experts' definitions of health are usually based on biophysical markers and often differ significantly from patients' assessments of their health, which are shaped by personal and cultural factors.[66] For example, one ethnographic study showed that while measures of physical health demonstrated clear improvements in the health of the Matsigenka indigenous people of the Peruvian Amazon over a thirty-year period, the Matsigenka themselves believed that their health had severely deteriorated over this time.[67] The Matsigenka understood health and well-being as comprising more than biophysical health. They viewed social changes such as permanent settlement and acculturation to mainstream Peruvian society as having a massive negative impact on their health.[68] This example illustrates a fundamental challenge when faced with different ways to assess a population's health.[69] If we privilege biophysical measures of health, we may devalue culturally meaningful definitions of health, and vice versa.

Another challenge is determining what causes improvements in a population's health. Measuring the effect of Barrio Adentro is difficult because Barrio Adentro emerged alongside other government programs to improve health and quality of life. We cannot isolate the effects of primary health care from the effects of other programs that probably improved people's health (such as literacy, education, housing, gender empowerment, nutrition, and employment programs). Community-run government soup kitchens (*casas de alimentación*) and government-subsidized grocery stores (Misión Mercal) provided poor and working-class Venezuelans with better access to nutritious food, which surely affected people's health.

Setting aside these concerns, we have seen improved biophysical measures of health and improved quality of life after the institution of Barrio Adentro and other social missions. Let us focus on life expectancy and infant mortality rates, the most commonly used indicators of a population's physical health. Already relatively high, Venezuelans' average life expectancy increased between 1990 and 2013 from 71 years to 75 years.[70] Infant mortality fell between 1990 and 2013 from 25 deaths per 1,000 births to 13 deaths per 1,000 births.[71] Venezuela's ranking in the United Nations Human Development

Index (which is tied to a range of quality of life measures) rose from its 1990s levels every year since Chávez took office until his death in 2013 (for a discussion of declining economic and health indicators after 2013, see my update in the conclusion).[72] And income inequality in Venezuela fell to one of the lowest levels in Latin America.[73]

Subjective assessments of health services and well-being were extremely favorable during Chávez's presidency. According to the United Nations Human Development Report for the period 2006–9, 80 percent of Venezuelans reported satisfaction with their standard of living.[74] And 90 percent reported satisfaction with their personal health—which is impressive, as only three countries worldwide claimed higher levels of satisfaction.[75] The same report found that 67 percent of Venezuelans were satisfied with their quality of health care, placing Venezuela high in world rankings.[76] Another survey conducted in 2008 confirmed the UN report's findings: in that study, 75 percent of Venezuelans reported satisfaction with walk-in clinics, 71 percent with hospital services.[77]

These data demonstrate that the personal narratives I present in this book represented the majority of Venezuelans' experiences and perspectives during this period. And like the Matsigenka, Venezuelans' assessments of their personal health do not directly map onto biophysical measures of population health. Yet subjective assessments of people's health and health care reveal volumes about how people experience their lives and their livelihoods in the context of their culture and their material realities. Understanding experiences of pleasure in medicine—in this case, understanding how engagements with government health care felt to people—is useful for reasons that have little to do with quantifiable measures of biophysical health. In order to understand the meanings that Venezuelans attach to their health and health care, we must move beyond numbers. We must listen to people's stories and interpret what they say and do in the context of their culture and history. Doing this requires different research methods—methods of ethnography that allow access to detailed and credible narratives of people's experiences.

METHODS

Field Site

I conducted fifteen months of ethnographic research across one of Caracas's vast municipalities, Libertador, spending most of my time in Santa Teresa, a

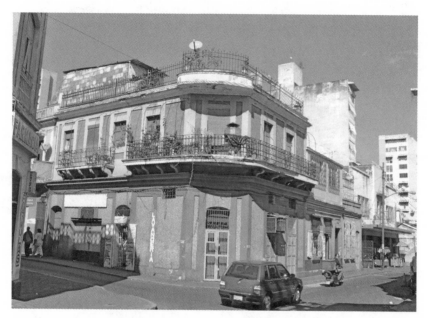

FIGURE 4. Street corner in Santa Teresa, 2006. Photo by the author.

smaller residential district.[78] Approximately 20,000 people lived in Santa Teresa in an area that comprises about thirty city blocks. The neighborhood is part of the *casco histórico,* the historic district of the city. Narrow sidewalks give way to boxy concrete apartment towers and ornate colonial buildings, the architecture reflecting different eras of urbanization (fig. 4). Heat from the sun radiated from cobblestone roads. Street vendors sold household goods, medicinal herbs, newspapers and legal codes, by-the-minute phone calls, and sweet milky *chicha.* There was little romance to the place. People gulped their coffees from plastic cups while standing at the bakery counter and walked the long way around the unkempt central plaza (fig. 5).

The neighborhood's socioeconomic standing depended on who you asked. Most residents described Santa Teresa as a working-class neighborhood (*trabajadora*), but depending on their class position, aspirations, and politics, some claimed it was a middle-class area (*clase media/media baja*), while others insisted it was a poor area (*pobre/humilde*). For example, a community health worker named Gabriella scoffed at the notion that Santa Teresa was middle class, claiming that a lot of poverty was hidden behind closed doors and that their multistory apartment blocks were in fact *ranchos verticales,* or vertical shanties. According to census data, the average monthly income of its

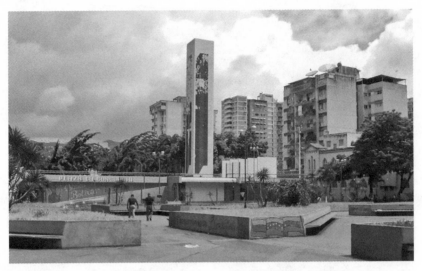

FIGURE 5. Santa Teresa's central plaza, Plaza La Concordia, 2006. Photo by the author.

population was slightly higher than the average for the municipality of Libertador as a whole, representing modest incomes within one of the poorest municipalities in the city.[79] Residents viewed their neighborhood as sharply divided between Chávez supporters and members of the conservative opposition, whereas in poorer neighboring areas there was more widespread support for the Chávez government.

Santa Teresa's heritage sites included the National Theater, the Basilica of Santa Teresa, and the home of the national liberation hero Simón Bolívar. But if you asked a resident about the area you would hear about its social problems rather than its attractions. Poverty, drug and alcohol abuse, dilapidated public spaces, prostitution, visible homelessness—these concerns troubled residents regardless of their class position or political persuasion.

No concern loomed larger than the fear of crime, glossed in the local dialect as *inseguridad* (insecurity). Santa Teresa's residents described the area as a "red zone" (*zona roja*). Homes featured elaborate security protocols to ward off inseguridad. Residents armored the windows of apartment buildings with burglar bars not only on the lower levels, but ten or fifteen stories high. One research participant's apartment could only be accessed by using five keys (including two just for the elevator) and getting past a security guard in the lobby. People from all over Caracas were preoccupied with inseguridad when I conducted fieldwork between 2006 and 2009. It was one of the only sentiments uniting a city deeply divided along socioeconomic and political fault lines. Never mind that the victims of violent crime were predominantly poor young men from barrios. The threat of inseguridad affected everyone. It was the awful background of daily life.

Before the first Barrio Adentro doctor began to work in Santa Teresa in 2004, the area did not have any government health clinics. If residents needed biomedical care, they went to a private practice doctor or traveled outside the neighborhood to a public hospital. By the time I was conducting fieldwork, there were two Barrio Adentro clinics (each with one doctor and nurse; one also offered dentistry services daily), one rehabilitation center in the final stages of construction, and a handful of government health promotion programs and other social missions such as Misión Negra Hipólita, a community-led homeless outreach program. Many other Barrio Adentro clinics had been built within walking distance or a short bus ride from the neighborhood.

Santa Teresa differed from the communities that have become de facto sites for research on urban Venezuela. Contemporary research on Venezuelan politics and social change has focused on the city's barrios.[80] Studying barrios makes sense because they were the main targets for social welfare interventions and had their own histories of autonomous community activism. But government projects like Barrio Adentro were instituted across the city, not only in the areas identified as barrios. I was interested in how the social and political transformations identified by other researchers unfolded in urban areas with diverse socioeconomic and political configurations.[81] This book examines how government health programs affected individuals from different types of communities. It explores how Santa Teresa's residents made sense of national discourses of popular participation and demarginalization and how they understood themselves and their neighborhood in comparison to the increasingly idealized barrios and their residents.

Research Methods

I spent fifteen months conducting ethnographic research, between May and July 2006 and between January 2008 and February 2009.[82] Immersive, in-depth fieldwork allowed me to collect detailed and credible information about people's experiences of health care. Fieldwork included extensive participant observation in each of Santa Teresa's Barrio Adentro clinics, observing hundreds of hours of doctor-patient and nurse-patient interactions.

I worked closely with the clinics' Health Committees, participating in outreach, community education, clinic administration, training, and political events with the neighborhood's team of volunteer health activists. I attended daily exercise classes and field trips with the local Grandparents Clubs. I collected fifty-seven detailed, semistructured interviews with patients, doctors, nurses, dentists, public health administrators, volunteer health workers, members of Grandparents Clubs, and community activists. Interviews occurred in respondents' homes, in clinics, or in a public space of the respondent's choosing (e.g., café, plaza, or community center). With the help of two Caraqueña college students working as my research assistants, I visited twenty-five other government clinics and hospitals across the city (some Barrio Adentro, some not) to understand the broader context of Venezuelan government medicine. My research assistants and I investigated popular healing sites and practices. I collected media and other documents from Venezuelan government ministries, medical institutions, activist networks, community centers, national daily newspapers, websites, the National Archives, and the National Statistics Institute.

Spatial segregation and political polarization shaped how people understood my presence as a foreign researcher. Poor barrios and neighborhoods like Santa Teresa were rarely visited by middle- and upper-class Caraqueños because of their reputations for violent crime.[83] The same was largely true of foreigners (e.g., the U.S. embassy in Caracas categorically prohibits U.S. personnel from entering many Libertador neighborhoods).[84] Because of this marked spatial segregation, people often assumed that my presence in their community signaled interest in their lives and that my research was inspired by a political commitment to social justice. Research participants, savvy about the international media's tendency to portray revolutionary Venezuela in overwhelmingly negative terms, viewed me as a conduit to communicate the benefits of government social programs to a global audience.

The way research participants perceived me facilitated establishing relationships of trust. Lilian and others members of Santa Teresa's Health Committees adopted me as a member of their group practically as soon as I met them. They included me in their work and took me to visit their counterparts in nearby barrios. Medical workers and activists encouraged me to document the conditions of government health facilities and the quantity of medications on hand to counter accusations by members of the right-wing opposition that these sites were nonfunctional. Fluid, candid conversations were the norm with Venezuelan medical professionals, medical students, community health workers, and patients.[85] People I got to know were as open with their critiques of government social programs as they were with their praise.

When people outside of Venezuela learn about this research, they sometimes wonder whether government officials controlled or managed my access to medical sites. They did not. I established initial contacts in Santa Teresa not through government officials but through U.S.-based scholars already studying Venezuelan health care. I gained access to other medical sites after introducing myself to health activists at public events. I visited dozens of government clinics and hospitals without prior permission or advance notice. My research assistants and I explained our interest in observing the facilities and were in all cases invited to visit and have conversations with staff members who had time to talk. As I explain in chapter 4, there was minimal or no government control over people's comings and goings in health care centers.

Journalists have published extensively about Venezuela and Chávez in the global media, but mainstream media reporting on life in Bolivarian Venezuela does not capture the full range of people's experiences, particularly those of historically marginalized people. Mainstream reporting tends to favor the points of view and narratives of historically privileged groups in Venezuela: the traditional political elite, the upper middle class, and the wealthy. Researchers analyzing ten years' worth of reporting by BBC News (the publicly owned British Broadcasting Corporation, the largest broadcaster in the world) found that of 304 news stories on Venezuela published on their website between 1998 and 2008, only three mentioned positive policies of the Chávez government.[86] Media misrepresentation of Venezuelan politics has extended to comparisons between Donald Trump and Hugo Chávez, though the two could hardly differ more in their personal identities or their politics. Robert Samet and Naomi Schiller, anthropologists of Venezuela, have commented on the absurdity of equating "an anti-capitalist who sought to build a type of socialism and a billionaire real estate developer who wants to further deregulate Wall Street."[87]

When media accounts downplay the concerns and experiences of a country's majority, ethnography can act as a corrective by offering detailed, credible accounts of daily life from the point of view of local actors. This book offers a unique set of observations of people engaging with leftist state projects. The people I knew were not naive: they did not think they were living with a perfect government or building a perfect society. But they were excited about the idea of building a more equitable society.

This book analyzes the positive meanings of government medicine in historical and cultural context. Each chapter explores a different aspect of health care to show what people gained from Venezuelan health programs beyond medicine. Chapter 2 analyzes the spatial significance of Barrio Adentro, revealing that building clinics in poor neighborhoods responded to a historical desire for community-based biomedicine and transformed the meaning of the neighborhoods. Chapter 3 focuses on doctor-patient encounters in neighborhood clinics. There I show that clinical interactions functioned as a microcosm of national politics because patients viewed doctors' expressions of care as symbolic of a government that finally cared about poor people. Chapter 4 explores how patients integrated new health services into their lives. People maintained agency with regard to how they used government health care in combination with popular healing traditions, in part because Venezuelan officials did not try to delegitimize alternative medicine. Chapters 5 and 6 focus on people engaged with government health programs in community (nonclinical) settings. Chapter 5 describes the experiences of volunteer health workers and members of exercise clubs for the elderly. For people who previously felt they had no stake in public life, participating in these programs produced a sense of empowerment related to revitalizing their communities. Chapter 6 analyzes why one government health program evoked displeasure rather than pleasure. Beneficiaries of a homeless outreach program who did not accept opportunities to rehabilitate themselves became a source of deep displeasure for community members because they threatened a utopian vision of social change that expected people to play an active role in their own empowerment. The conclusion summarizes how government health programs enacted feelings of empowerment and sociopolitical belonging. It considers what the future holds for people's experiences of health care in Venezuela amid ongoing political and economic precarity.

TWO

Moving Medicine Inside the Barrio

PEOPLE'S NARRATIVES OF HEALTH CARE before and after Barrio Adentro reveal that the spatial reorganization of government medicine responded to historical desires and changed the meanings of their neighborhoods. Long stigmatized for endangering residents' lives through violence and state neglect, barrios and other poor neighborhoods took on new significance as places that could be productive of health. In revolutionary Venezuela, moving medicine inside the neighborhood effected positive transformations for communities beyond improved access to medicine.

Many Venezuelans said that before Barrio Adentro the best hope many poor people had to see a doctor inside their neighborhoods was to pray that the beloved doctor-saint José Gregorio Hernández would appear to them in a vision. José Gregorio provides cultural context for understanding the political significance of the government assigning doctors to live and work in poor neighborhoods. Before discussing health care under Chávez, let us consider how a doctor known for making house calls to poor Caracas neighborhoods has been Venezuela's most popular saint for over a century.

A VENEZUELAN SAINT AND THE HUNGER FOR HEALTH CARE

I knew I had stumbled across an important feature of Venezuelans' relationship with medicine my first week in Caracas when I noticed a street vendor selling religious statues of a man wearing a doctor's white coat. I cupped a little replica in my hands, curious about the symbolic fusion of biomedicine and faith.[1] The plaster figure represented a Venezuelan doctor named José

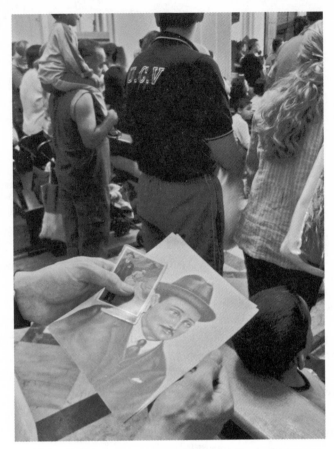

FIGURE 6. Images of doctor-saint José Gregorio Hernández at a mass
honoring his birth, Iglesia de la Candelaria, 2008. Photo by the author.

Gregorio Hernández. He skyrocketed to spiritual celebrity in the early 1900s
when people claimed that he performed healing miracles in the afterlife. He
became the country's most beloved popular saint, revered not only by
Catholics but also by practitioners of the possession cult of María Lionza.[2]
Images of the anachronistic mustachioed doctor were ubiquitous in Caracas:
painted on the sides of buses; displayed in homes and hospitals, on devotional
cards in wallets, and on the covers of history magazines at the newsstand; and
as figurines sold outside churches and in healing shops (fig. 6). After noticing
him once, I saw him everywhere.

José Gregorio was a beloved public figure even before he became known
as a miraculous healer. He was one of the country's first physicians and

scientists when biomedicine was gaining prominence in the Americas. José Gregorio studied medicine in France in the 1890s, bringing home to Venezuela the country's first microscope and blood pressure gauge.[3] He headed the laboratory of experimental physiology and bacteriology at the Universidad Central de Venezuela in Caracas and trained medical students.[4] Being a founding father of Venezuelan medicine gave José Gregorio prestige and authority, but he won the hearts of poor people by caring for them in their neighborhoods.

A deeply religious Catholic, José Gregorio popularized biomedicine among nonelite Venezuelans by practicing it as a vocation and treating poor Caraqueños in their homes free of charge. He gained renown for traveling to poor neighborhoods, making house calls, and even buying medication for his patients. Although Venezuelans across class and racial divides believe in José Gregorio, he is particularly important for poor Venezuelans. Because of his good works, he was known as *el médico de los pobres,* "the doctor of the poor." This association distinguished him from other doctors of his era and contributed to his status as a divine healer. His followers were devastated when a car struck and killed him when he was making a house call in 1919. The day of his funeral, a crowd of thirty thousand people—one-third of the population of Caracas at the time—filled the streets to accompany his casket to the cemetery.[5] His popularity continues unabated today. In 2014, the Catholic Church received over eight hundred separate testimonials of miracles performed by José Gregorio as evidence for his canonization.[6]

Nearly every Caraqueño I asked told me a personal story about *el santo médico* (the doctor-saint) and his mystical healing powers. People said he appeared to them in visions. Often he cured the sick while they slept. A domestic worker and single mother from Santa Teresa named Paola told me this story:

> My parents used to tell me he was a very humanitarian doctor: he gave everything he had to cure patients. He was on the way to see a sick person when he had his accident, you know? . . . He was like something divine, he was like a saint. . . . I still remember when my daughter had an operation in the Pérez Carreño [Hospital], she told me that a person visited her dressed in black and wearing a small black hat. This was Doctor José Gregorio. When her doctor came to see her before the operation—he thought she wouldn't live—I put a picture of Doctor José Gregorio right next to her bed. And my daughter saw the picture and said, "Mamá, look, that's who came to see me last night!" She was eight years old.

Carina, a self-described "fanatic" of Barrio Adentro from Santa Teresa, joked that "even the atheists" in Venezuela believe in José Gregorio. She told me about her mother's encounter with the doctor-saint.

> My mother says when she was pregnant with my oldest brother . . . she was at the point of giving birth, okay? . . . Her parents took her to the Maternidad [Maternity Hospital], and this doctor with a little mustache delivered her baby and she thought he looked like José Gregorio. It turned out she was just dreaming. . . . [But in the dream] the doctor calmed her, saying, "No girl, tranquila, because everything's going to be fine." She thought, "[I was visited by] José Gregorio Hernández." But then she said, "No, this was just a dream I had of being in the hospital, what do I know?" But when she actually gave birth, she told me that the exact same baby she'd seen in the dream turned out to be her son. And I believe her because my mom is not a [religious] fanatic at all, you know.

Every person I asked could cite the details of José Gregorio's biography as "el médico de los pobres." For example, Carina, whose mother's dream of José Gregorio presaged the healthy delivery of her oldest brother, said:

> He represents the kind of human being we wish everyone could be, I think it's something like that, no? Because of his history: he was a super generous man, you know? He took care of poor people, he never charged them money, he would give them their remedies, and as a result he was very beloved. He was very beloved, and this humanity, I believe that people yearn for that humanity, no? They don't want that to disappear, you see?

Echoing Carina's knowledge of José Gregorio's importance as a model for Venezuelans, a nursing student from Santa Teresa named Ana said:

> He is very important because he was a very modest doctor [un doctor muy humilde]. He didn't charge anyone for medical consultations, he took care of his people, and furthermore, he would gift them with medicines. This man was so modest, so humble, that regardless of the hour he would get out of bed to go to a sick person's home. The truth is he was a very special person, and we should remember him as a humanistic human being. Doctors today should emulate him.

A religious icon and Chávez-era government health care have more in common than we might initially assume. Since the early 1900s doctor-saint José Gregorio symbolically substituted for a state that promised medical access to the people but never fully delivered on that promise. We can interpret José Gregorio's popularity as a response to the lack of health care that poor people experienced. But more important than simply reflecting a desire for medicine, José Gregorio symbolizes access to a particular style of medicine that has long been inaccessible to marginalized Caraqueños. He points to a hunger for a model of health care that is local, caring, and focused on the poor and marginalized. The figure of José Gregorio underlines the importance of providing community-based medical care regardless of people's ability to pay. His popularity communicates Venezuelans' desires that doctors work in poor neighborhoods and that they display other attributes associated with *el médico de los pobres,* such as expressing care for poor patients and a vocation for service.

THE SIGNIFICANCE OF MOVING MEDICINE INSIDE THE BARRIO

This chapter and the next show that Barrio Adentro responded to a long-standing desire for a local and caring form of medicine. Mara Gomez, who directed the health department for Caracas's Libertador Municipality, told me that the idea of systematically sending doctors into barrios was inspired by José Gregorio. According to Gomez, government researchers conducting fieldwork in municipality barrios observed the preponderance of José Gregorio iconography in people's homes and interpreted it as evidence that "people needed and wanted a doctor in their homes and their neighborhoods."[7] Barrio Adentro began as a pilot project run by Libertador's health department in 2002 with a few dozen doctors. The following year, Chávez expanded Barrio Adentro into a national program and made it a cornerstone of the government's social welfare programs, or missions (*misiones*). In Libertador Municipality (one of five municipalities in Caracas) over five hundred Barrio Adentro clinics opened between 2002 and 2008.

When people talked about the significance of Barrio Adentro, they often focused on the importance of doctors being accessible in poor neighborhoods. Mariángela explained the effects of Barrio Adentro in spatial terms.

> I'll speak first about what's happening at the national level and that is that the Venezuelan doctors, I don't know why, but they haven't wanted to integrate themselves, but you'll see that the Cuban doctors are spread out across the entire country: there isn't the smallest corner of Alto Apure or Amazonas [in Venezuela] where they are not offering their solidarity, their medicine, all

the way to the indigenous communities of the Wayúu, the Piaroa . . . all the way to the very top of the *cerro* Petare [in eastern Caracas]! The people [there] have told me, "Look, señora, here if we don't have a car and we have to get a patient to medical care at 11:00 or 12:00 at night, they die on us," and more than one has died because the transports only run until a certain hour. So the miracle that here you have right beside your house a doctor, this is a blessing of God, and this is thanks to the Cuban-Venezuelan agreement, you know?

Mariángela evoked imagery of an animated map of the country with doctors and medical services flowing from economic and political centers to peripheral zones. Her description of Barrio Adentro as a miraculous place where a doctor is right next door resonates with people's descriptions of the beloved doctor-saint José Gregorio Hérnandez. However, rather than the result of divine intervention, Barrio Adentro is a "blessing of God . . . thanks to the Cuban-Venezuelan agreement." Mariángela claimed that recently placed Cuban doctors were more willing to work in marginalized communities than Venezuelan doctors, a claim I heard many times during fieldwork that revealed speakers' perceptions of spatialized social inequalities in the country.

"Deep inside the Barrios"

In the run-up to Christmas 2008 I spent the day with community activists and medical workers in the hills of a barrio in Catia. This is a sprawling region in western Caracas where families built their homes, sidewalks, and staircases into steep hillsides (fig. 7). Adapted four-wheel-drive trucks, or *camionetas,* traversed uneven roads, ferrying residents between their homes and the main streets below. Wilmer, a community activist I knew from city meetings and events, brought me to his neighborhood's Barrio Adentro clinic. I sat with Wilmer, two community health workers, a Venezuelan nurse, and the Cuban doctor in the living room of a home that neighbors had been lending the community to use as a clinic for the past five years. We talked for hours. Meanwhile, patients circulated through the clinic, sitting on couches and joining us mid-conversation. We drank dark sweet coffee and enjoyed holiday *hallacas,* savory-sweet tamales of meat, olives, and raisins wrapped in bright green banana leaves.

Research participants said theirs was a long-established barrio and that the home hosting this clinic was over sixty years old. They were at pains to communicate that this was not a barrio characterized by extreme poverty

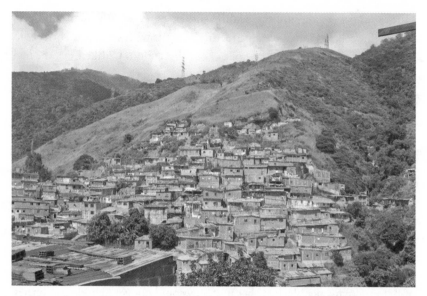

FIGURE 7. Barrio of Catia, 2008. Photo by the author.

(*pobreza extrema*). Many residents attended college and worked in the formal economy. In spite of this, before Barrio Adentro there was nowhere in the neighborhood to access free health care and people suffered. Luis, a middle-aged community health worker, leaned in excitedly to tell me this history. Luis's personal style—his close-cropped hair and bright polo shirt tucked into starched blue jeans—telegraphed his earnestness. He described himself as a formerly apathetic person whose initiation into leftist activism after Chávez's election was like "being born again." Luis explained:

> Before all this, there were hospitals that would see you at 8:00 in the morning, but in order to be seen you had to go there at 5:00 in the morning and get in line to take a number. If that hospital was able to attend to 40 patients, in the line there might be 100, right? They would give out numbers from 1 to 40, and beyond that, independent of what problem you had, they wouldn't see you. . . .
>
> Here, many people died, just in trying to get down to the transportation, you know? There just wasn't transportation, and then, if they could even get to the hospitals, who would take care of these people? The hospitals were totally, totally congested [*colapsado*], it was hellish. Then, the Barrio Adentro network was born. . . . [T]ruly, from our point of view, health has advanced considerably. These primary care [clinics] are here so the hospitals don't come to a standstill, so the hospitals don't become even more congested.

Mireya, another community health worker, agreed with many of Luis's points. She relaxed into a couch, greeting patients with smiles and brief conversations while jumping in and out of our discussion. Unlike Luis, she had been involved in leftist activism for years, since grade school when she would sneak over to the Central University to join the student protests. When Luis began a point-by-point comparison of leftist governments in Latin America, Mireya gently suggested we pause the political discourse to better enjoy our hallacas. When she saw an opening in the conversation, she said:

> Barrio Adentro came to the unattended areas, you see? To the people that truly didn't have medical attention. The name says it all: Inside the Barrio, for those people who didn't have the option of going to a clinic and had to struggle to access the hospitals. At the start of Barrio Adentro, more and more people came to the clinic; they got medical attention 24 hours a day, and well, it improved their quality of life.

Before, "many people died" because they could not get to hospitals or they were not in line early enough to see a doctor. Now, the doctor and nurse staffed the barrio's clinic in the morning and made house calls in the afternoon—the expected practice for Barrio Adentro community clinics. Wilmer confirmed this.

> Regarding the health network that is inside, inside, inside, *deep* inside the barrios, truly its functionality has been excellent, and people's acceptance of it has been fantastic. There are clinics, good clinics. People don't have any reason to leave their sector in order to get their blood pressure taken or to get treatments, to get stitches or whatever, because they have everything there at their fingertips.

Wilmer and Luis exuded enthusiasm when they talked about the spatial significance of Barrio Adentro clinics. In daily practice, staff at the clinics spent most of their time on preventive care, treating common colds, and monitoring chronic health problems. Hypertension, asthma, and diabetes became the rote, predictable diagnoses. In my observations the medical work in Barrio Adentro was repetitive, often mundane. In a cultural context in which access to medicine was longer established, these clinics probably would have faded into the background as unremarked fixtures of the urban landscape. Yet Venezuelan activists, health workers, and patients repeatedly emphasized that localizing access to health care made the difference between life and death.

Lisbeth, whose chronic asthma sent her to the clinic in the middle of our interview, shared her medical history with me. Everyone in the clinic knew her health background. She said:

> Since Barrio Adentro began, I don't go to the hospital now like I did before. Before I used to go to the hospital and I had to wait in line, [but] you know that an asthmatic can't wait. Since Barrio Adentro started here in the sector, I don't go to the hospital for anything anymore, instead I just come up here to the walk-in clinic. At night or whatever time it is, they see me; and I have received very good care. Everything that they have done here with regard to health has been really great, for myself and for my children. [Before], for every type of medicine, I had to buy the medicine. Now I hardly buy any medicine, they give it to me here.

We discussed her first experience with Barrio Adentro.

LISBETH: Well, I'll tell you that I got pneumonia. Pneumonia with bronchitis. Well, it was horrible and I was dying. I went to the hospital, I went every day. I was so thin, of course, and afraid. . . . They told me, "Go see the Cuban doctors, they are giving good medical care." And thank God . . .

AMY: Who said that?

LISBETH: [People from] here in the community, because I was completely disoriented.

AMY: Ah, OK, so you didn't know [about Barrio Adentro]?

LISBETH: No. And Ms. Janeth [the nurse] came down with the doctor who was here before, to treat me at my house because I was feeling like I couldn't get out of bed. I didn't move or anything, all the medicine that the hospital gave me was for nothing. They have the patience to come down to one's house, to walk even to where one wouldn't [normally] walk to attend to you. The care has been very good.

Luis added his personal narrative, revealing his concern that ongoing controversy over Barrio Adentro obscured its manifest benefits.

> Truly [Barrio Adentro] is greatly satisfying for all of the communities. I am one of those cases, no? When Barrio Adentro arrived here with Dr. Ivan and Dr. Nelson, my mom got sick. She got very sick due to her blood pressure. She had already had treatment for blood pressure for a few years, [but] the treatment hadn't worked very well and she had a setback, in 2002 or 2003. Barrio Adentro arrived, and those were the years in which the public health system was more bogged down due to strikes and boycotts on the part of the doctors and the entire union. Everything was completely broken down. So

Barrio Adentro had arrived, and they treated her. If they hadn't given her that treatment, it wouldn't have done any good to take her to the closest medical center, with the little money we had, [and] today I wouldn't be able to tell you that she is healthy. That is one of many lives saved.

Although there are many who don't want to recognize this reality. A reality that we have right in front of us. That woman would not be here if Barrio Adentro hadn't arrived. We have had experiences with the doctors in the hospitals, in the clinics, even in the Military Hospital; they are all very good for sure. But since Barrio Adentro arrived the craziness of getting up at 5:00 in the morning with someone of that age is eliminated, you have to take that into account. Maybe with money to take a taxi and get to the closest center and I would have had to take her in a bus; that is a lot for someone of that age. One of the benefits that Barrio Adentro gives us is not having to take a person out at 6:00 in the morning to a bus, in a jeep, or whatever.

I have evidence that Barrio Adentro has truly given a great level of satisfaction to the community. And we should continue defending it.

Some conversations that I observed, like this one, have the feeling of a testimonial. Right-wing antagonism directed at Chávez-era social programs affected how supporters talked about Barrio Adentro. For Luis, locating health care in poor neighborhoods was obvious, yet it was also something he felt he had to justify and protect. Thus stories of pleasure and satisfaction were not simply commentaries on experiences inside a clinic. They represented local responses to acrimonious national and international debates about the value of the Bolivarian Revolution. Research participants instructed me to return to the United States and share their narratives, hoping that their stories would undermine unfavorable mainstream reporting on Venezuelan society under Chávez.[8] Near the end of my visit that day, Luis said:

Look, Amy, I want you to know something, so that you can say it in your country, and so that you can say it where it needs to be said. For fifty years we lived without a public health system in Venezuela. We never had one. The public health systems have always been dependent upon the *alcaldías* [mayors' offices], on the government, as well as on some other administrative bodies. In the Constitution that was approved by our presi—, by our people, we all approved this Constitution: it was established in the year 1999, for the first time. In Article 84, the creation of a national public health system. From that moment on, since the Constitution of 1999, until now in 2008, we have been fighting, okay? Against all adversity, in order to create a national public health system. Because here, in Venezuela, what still prevails is the private system that fed off of the public system during all these years, which is the reason why many people agree on the idea that it is better to privatize health because the private clinics work well. That is a fallacy. That is a lie. It is the biggest lie that a Venezuelan could tell.

Luis emphasized the people's role in creating Barrio Adentro by focusing on the fact that ordinary Venezuelans were instrumental in writing the constitution that established universal health care as a basic right, correcting himself when he first attributed the achievement to Chávez. His ability to cite the specific article that guaranteed access to health care was nothing special; many people began studying and memorizing legal documents at this time as a form of political participation that the revolutionary government encouraged. When Luis claimed that "the private system fed off the public one" for many years, he was referring to the widely held belief that doctors working in both government hospitals and private clinics (a very common practice) diverted equipment and supplies from public centers to their private offices. In framing private medicine as parasitical, Luis was undercutting claims that private medicine is superior.

Locating Barrio Adentro clinics in neighborhoods that previously had no government health presence carried political meaning for residents. Luis explained that Barrio Adentro made invisible people visible and integrated them into society. In other words, he argued that beyond providing tangible medical benefits, Barrio Adentro effected sociopolitical changes for poor and working-class people. Referring to people with disabilities, Luis said:

> A lot of people from this community didn't know that we had people with a disability here, right? That is, until Barrio Adentro came and was able to provide attention to the most needy and get to the most remote places, and those people came out, right? Like they say, they popped up. And we should take notice of them, independently of the problems they could have or their disability. They are part of society, they are citizens like we all are, and therefore they have social rights the same as the rest of us. So that has been one of the important things—that in one way or another people who were truly stuck inside four walls have been incorporated into society.

Luis's comments about empowering people with disabilities could pertain to the entire community. By going into "the most remote places" in the city or, as Mireya said earlier, "the unattended areas," providing constitutionally guaranteed services, Barrio Adentro formally recognized their residents as "part of society" deserving the same rights as other citizens.

Although clearly excited about Barrio Adentro's transformation of poor neighborhoods, patients and community health workers were aware of the program's limitations. Luis might seem to have a romantic or even naive view, but he was the person in this group who seemed most interested in discussing the problems that continued to threaten people's health. He listed ongoing health needs in the barrio and suggested his own solutions. For example, Luis wanted a fleet of vehicles to take patients to specialized medical facilities, and he wanted to reclaim and repurpose abandoned buildings to house more social services. Research participants were quick to point out that health threats abounded in the barrio that could not be addressed by medical initiatives. For example, Wilmer had to leave our interview early to attend a meeting about a rapidly growing crisis involving uncollected rubbish piling up across the neighborhood.

The Spatial Importance of Doctors' Work

Viki and Katerina, college students in their early twenties, associated the presence and absence of clinics in poor neighborhoods with the personal qualities of doctors. Like many people I interviewed, they expressed pleasure that the Barrio Adentro program was building clinics in poor neighborhoods, but they pointed out that this dynamic depended on the political will of doctors as well as the government. Our interview took place in Katerina's apartment in Santa Teresa. Katerina is the daughter of Lilian, a well-known health activist in Santa Teresa. Viki lived in the same building and had firsthand experience with Venezuelan doctors in hospital placements as a nursing student at the prestigious Universidad Central de Venezuela. Katerina had worked with me briefly as a research assistant, and together we interviewed Viki, though Katerina found herself speaking as well.

> AMY: What is the difference between Barrio Adentro and other systems of public health?
>
> VIKI: Look, there's a big difference because Barrio Adentro has integrated itself in a very special way that is aimed at the patient. In other words, Barrio Adentro is a very profound public health system because it is in the barrios, whereas doctors previously did not go to the barrios. Now, Barrio Adentro is indeed including all these areas, you see?
>
> KATERINA: In other words, it is including the excluded [los excluidos].
>
> VIKI: Yes, exactly. Including the excluded. I mean, the excluded don't have to come down here. Right up there we have Barrio Adentro and with specialist doctors, those with medical specialties.

My open-ended question about what made Barrio Adentro special elicited a response that focused on the spatial significance of the program. Viki and Katerina explained the importance of local access to health care in terms of convenience and efficiency: people can see specialists right where they live.

Viki and Katerina claimed that the spatial aspects of health care shaped social and political relations. In addition to achieving the pragmatic goal of making medicine more accessible, establishing clinics in barrios effected sociopolitical change by "including the excluded." The term "los excluidos" refers to people or communities who have been historically marginalized from formal participation in Venezuelan politics, economic life, and educational opportunities. From this conversation we can glean the degree to which space influenced one's position in the social hierarchy. If someone lived in a barrio, then by default she was excluded in key ways, not fully integrated into the social, political, and economic life of the city. According to Viki and Katerina, a program like Barrio Adentro addressed this history of exclusion. By providing poor communities with clinics and doctors, Barrio Adento resignified these spaces and their residents by including them in a regime of care and formally recognizing them as people who mattered to the state. Barrio Adentro was doing more than filling a gap in access to medicine. It was also identifying marginalized places and peoples as deserving of recognition and social inclusion. If we understand this, it is easier to understand people's emotional responses to the program.

Viki and Katerina reiterated the clinical and sociopolitical importance of putting clinics in poor areas.

VIKI: Without a doubt, they created these [Barrio Adentro] clinics and distributed these clinics in neighborhoods that truly need them.

KATERINA: [Before,] many doctors didn't want to go to these places, because [sarcastically], "Ay, no, I am a *doctor*! *Please,* me, go all the way over *there*?"

VIKI: The reality is they did not want to work with this type of population. The population that's there, of low . . . , of low income, you know? They didn't want to do it. They didn't want to, they didn't want to, they didn't want to work there: not due to a fear of violent crime [*inseguridad*] and not for any other reason. Just because they didn't want to deal with this type of people.

KATERINA: Girlfriend, the thing is, you have to have a vocation to do this. If you are a doctor you have to take care of everyone, all the way down to the puppy you find dying in the street.

My fieldwork revealed that many Barrio Adentro patients desired regular access to medical services. They viewed the placement of clinics and doctors in barrios and other poor neighborhoods as necessary to guarantee access to medical care when needed. For Katerina, this issue was personal. She told me that when she was fourteen, her father took her to every public hospital in the city trying to get medical attention for her acute abdominal pain. She described the experience as one of being *peloteando,* kicked like a soccer ball from hospital to hospital. This was a common experience among people who relied on the state's medical services. Other people talked of being denied care and bouncing from one hospital to another because of overcrowding.

Yet this discussion extended beyond simply affirming the pragmatic logic of putting medical care in community settings. Viki and Katerina commented on the negative stigma that followed barrio residents. They criticized doctors, who have a moral obligation "to take care of everyone," for expressing fear and disgust when asked to work in barrios, for barrio residents. They interpreted doctors' absence from poor neighborhoods as evidence of contempt for the poor and as betraying the Venezuelan idea of how a doctor should behave. Research participants knew that Barrio Adentro hired Cubans because so few Venezuelan physicians applied to work for the program after a nationwide call went out.[9] Though patients acknowledged that barrio spaces could be physically difficult to access and posed a higher risk of violent crime, they argued that the lack of Venezuelan doctors in these areas was due to their disinterest in the poor. Hence Katerina's comment that in order to be a good doctor, one had to have a vocation for service. Her idea of a good doctor resonates with popular imaginaries of José Gregorio Hernández.

Resignifying Stigmatized Spaces

Analyzing the sociopolitical significance of clinic locations helps explain why Barrio Adentro elicited pleasure from patients. In a context of marked spatial segregation along class lines, in which middle- and upper-class Venezuelans were unlikely to ever visit poor Caracas neighborhoods, the symbolic significance of having medical professionals live and work inside poor communities was huge. Patients' insistence that doctors travel to and live in poor areas challenged long-standing inequalities between marginalized and privileged social groups in Caracas. The pleasure that patients expressed about having access to Barrio Adentro medical care reflected these political changes. By resignifying barrio spaces and changing what it meant to live in a poor neighborhood, Barrio Adentro offered benefits beyond medicine.

Barrio Adentro programs were intended to improve the status of poor neighborhoods and actively sought to communicate these extramedical effects to the public. Through language and other symbols, government officials reframed existing understandings of barrios and barrio residents. From its beginnings in 2002, the health program was discussed as a project promoting equal access to care in spatial terms, evident from the program's name. In a country beset by striking social inequalities, instituting a health program called Inside the Barrio makes a political statement about which communities merit attention and resources. Symbolic features of Barrio Adentro, such as the iconic architecture of the eight-sided red brick clinics, differed from every other aspect of the built environment. They were unmistakable symbols of government care and social change that visually stood out from the landscape, marking poor neighborhoods as capable of attending to people's health. This was important in a city like Caracas where many communities and their residents experienced stigma on a daily basis.

Barrio Adentro changed neighborhoods physically, and it changed how people used them by building clinics, providing health services, and reclaiming space for pro-social purposes. Poor neighborhoods quite literally became more therapeutic spaces after the institution of Barrio Adentro. For some zones, this change was dramatic, as in Santa Teresa, which had no public health presence prior to the arrival of a Barrio Adentro doctor in 2004. These changes were not top-down processes led by the state. They were bottom-up practices of space making because the government relied on community activists to identify disused spaces and oversee the construction teams building clinics.[10]

In densely populated urban areas, community health workers established new clinics by repurposing government offices, using residents' homes, or taking over abandoned buildings. Participants in Grandparents Clubs used public school courtyards and neighborhood plazas to perform daily exercises, staking out these spaces for leisurely socializing and community well-being. Government officials organized with activists to host *jornadas de salud* (health fairs) in neighborhood plazas, repurposing public spaces for health promotion. Public spaces such as parks and plazas were generally not considered healthful or safe, so offering health services in them was not an expected or neutral act. Drawing people into public spaces to exercise or receive medical care remade the meaning of these places.

In the process of providing health services, government institutions promoted barrios and their residents as deserving the state's care. When for decades a doctor's visit was something that only the elite could be assured of getting whenever they wanted, having an easily accessible doctor in one's neighborhood signified an opportunity for empowerment. The spatial logic of Barrio Adentro involved residents of historically marginalized zones of the city in relations of belonging with an oil-rich state from which they had long felt excluded.

THREE

Clinical Intimacies as Macropolitics

PATIENTS AT BARRIO ADENTRO CLINICS took immense pleasure in the way doctors treated poor people. Perhaps more than any other feature of new health programs, people valued the intimacy of doctor-patient encounters in neighborhood clinics. Patients interpreted eye contact, physical closeness, and informal speech as expressions of care and egalitarian solidarity on the part of doctors—and the state that employed them. I show that clinical interactions constituted a microcosm of national politics, as patients judged the revolutionary state's efforts to address sociopolitical inequalities by the bodily dispositions of its medical workers. For people who reported a history of feeling marginalized by elite, emotionally distant physicians, feeling cared for by Barrio Adentro doctors was deeply satisfying because it produced a sense of sociopolitical belonging.

DOCTORS WITH "THE SPIRIT OF BARRIO ADENTRO"

A quiet morning was unfolding in the small Barrio Adentro clinic in Santa Teresa. Patients sat in a semicircle in the front room, watching TV and waiting to see the doctor. I stood in the exam room that held the clinic's medicines and vaccines, chatting with Alejandra, the clinic's nurse, and Magdalena, a community health worker. Dr. Cardenas stomped out of his office, red-faced and upset. He wore his standard outfit: a button-down shirt haphazardly tucked into baggy slacks and a fanny pack stuffed with prescription pads and medical instruments. Neglecting the typical Caraqueño greeting of a kiss on each cheek, he thrust a paper and pen at me and ordered, "Write today's date, October 7, 2008, write 'Caracas,' then write that you are an anthropologist,

47

and you observed me treating the patients here with excellent care [*tratamiento excelente*]." As he left the room, I raised my eyebrows at Alejandra for an explanation. "Don't worry about it," she replied. "The Cuban doctors are staying out of it, and you should too—you don't need to get involved."

Dr. Cardenas was angry. Santa Teresa residents and Barrio Adentro community health workers had collected signatures and lodged a formal complaint (*denuncia*) with the municipal health department, asking to have him replaced. This drama revealed intense animosity between the doctor and his patients and community health workers. To go to such lengths to have a doctor replaced suggested that he violated deeply held medical values or expectations. In the United States, such a response might be prompted by gross negligence on the part of the practicing physician.

I tried to learn what Cardenas had done to elicit this reaction. At first the complaint puzzled me. Alejandra, who previously worked as a surgical nurse in the well-regarded Military Hospital, assured me that Cardenas, a Venezuelan doctor, had decades of experience and delivered sound medical treatment. Even those who complained about him acknowledged that he was a well-trained physician.

The more I inquired, the more I understood that people's discontent with Cardenas was not caused by acts of medical incompetence or by clear-cut violations of medical ethics. People did not even give the same reason for having presented the denuncia. One person claimed the complaint took shape after Cardenas left the clinic unstaffed to take an unapproved holiday. This certainly created an inconvenience as patients had to walk to another clinic nearby, but clinics commonly closed on short notice for a variety of reasons (including holidays). Lilian cited his practice of prescribing homeopathic remedies in conjunction with pharmaceutical treatments as a factor contributing to the denuncia. However, this practice was not unusual in Venezuelan biomedical settings and was in keeping with local practices of medical pluralism. Another person explained that the denuncia hinged on Cardenas not making house calls or extending his clinic hours beyond the time he was required to work. This critique was closest to a breach of practice, although neighborhood residents were themselves unclear about whether making house calls and extending office hours were required of Barrio Adentro doctors or were merely expected because this was what the Cuban doctors did.

Beyond all this, Cardenas seemed to breed resentment because he did not embody people's expectations of a caring Barrio Adentro doctor. People complained that he did not spend enough time talking to patients or explaining treatments, and he did not look patients in the eyes. I observed 125 doctor-patient interactions with Dr. Cardenas over a two-month period in 2008. During this period, I found Dr. Cardenas's bedside manner gruff: he rarely smiled and did not engage in small talk, which was unusual for people in this setting. However, that did not strike me as strange compared to busy doctors I encountered in the United States. For this reason, I failed to notice behaviors that locals interpreted as highly undesirable in a doctor. As we spent time together, Cardenas began to tell me what he thought of his job. When he was out of earshot of others, he complained that as a graduate of a prestigious medical school he was overqualified for the position of community doctor. He belittled the apartment above the clinic that the government provided for his family (fig. 8). He criticized the residents of the neighborhood for expecting too much from him and for not working hard enough to improve their lives. Cardenas confided that he hoped to find a job in Spain, where doctors were appreciated and paid better. One day I noticed a typed sign in the clinic waiting room, advising patients on how to speak to the doctor. It read, "How easy is it to say: 'please'; 'thank you'; 'can you do me the favor of . . .'" Even if Cardenas was not sharing his opinions with anyone else, he communicated his distaste for the role of community doctor and the people in the neighborhood through his actions.

The effort to oust Dr. Cardenas from his job forced me to recognize the intangible, deeply felt values that underlay people's assumptions about what made a good doctor in this cultural context. What upset people about Dr. Cardenas's behavior was not limited to problems accessing treatments. He offended people by displaying behaviors and mannerisms that made him seem uncaring and disinterested.

Magdalena communicated her thoughts about Cardenas many times over the course of my fieldwork. Sometimes her views took the form of a grumbled aside; at other times they spilled out in an impassioned soliloquy about medicine. More than anyone else I knew, Magdalena helped me clarify the logic that guided people's judgments about doctors. She helped me see that people's emotionally charged responses to doctors' behaviors were important because a doctor represented much more than an individual healer or even a philosophical approach to medicine. In Bolivarian Venezuela, doctors represented entire political and economic systems, and patients' relationships with doctors could symbolize their relationship with the Venezuelan state.

Magdalena lived and breathed Barrio Adentro. Described by her friends as unassuming and humble (*humilde*), Magdalena was the only Caraqueña

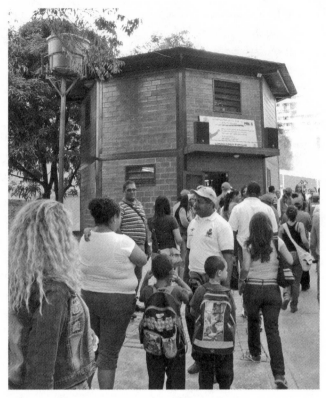

FIGURE 8. Barrio Adentro neighborhood clinic (second story intended for doctor's residence), 2008. Photo by the author.

I knew under the age of seventy who seemed not to care about her appearance. A statuesque woman of Afro-Venezuelan descent, her default uniform was a pair of baggy sweatpants and a loose T-shirt. She never wore makeup and did not dye her salt-and-pepper hair, rejecting social norms in which maintaining feminine beauty was assumed to be a national duty.[1] In addition to working full-time as a government social promoter (a position similar to a social worker with a focus on health issues), at fifty-eight Magdalena was taking night classes offered by the Chávez government to make up for the fact that her adoptive parents took her out of school after fourth grade. Our meetings in the clinic included up to an hour of English practice, with Magdalena painstakingly pronouncing each word of the current lesson in her *Misión Ribas* workbook for my approval. Participating in the educational mission and practicing her faith (evangelical Christianity) were Magdalena's two great passions after health activism. Any given day, Magda would invite me to several government-sponsored health events that she was organizing or participating in. She was never without a small sheath of medical *informes,* requests she prepared for residents who needed a special drug or medical device. As part of her job, she walked the city center hand delivering the informes to different institutions, including the presidential palace.

Magdalena was outspoken in her beliefs about what made a good doctor. Once while walking to the Metro and sipping cans of sugary soda, Magda described the doctor who previously held Cardenas's position, a Cuban woman named Misleidis. Magdalena started doing community work with this doctor; they would make house calls together (*hacer terreno*). Magda said there was one patient who was very sick. She was confined to bed and didn't want to eat or even try to stand up. Misleidis cajoled her into accepting help and convinced the woman to attend bailoterapia classes and work with a physical therapist. The sick woman ended up getting better and in the end, expressed deep appreciation for the help. Magdalena told me the patient was an "escualido" (squalid one, a derogatory term used to describe right-wing opponents of the Chávez government). Magdalena emphasized that Misleidis went to great trouble to heal a woman who was probably opposed to Barrio Adentro and to the presence of Cuban doctors in Venezuela. She praised Misleidis for helping patients even when medications were unavailable and for being willing to leave her house in the middle of a meal if she learned someone needed her. As we navigated sidewalks crowded with street vendors and newsstands, Magdalena paused for dramatic emphasis, saying, "*That* is Barrio Adentro. It is about a feeling, a love for the people!" She thumped her chest for emphasis, suggesting that the love doctors held for patients was located deep in their bodies.

"The doctor who's here now, he does not have the spirit of Barrio Adentro," Magdalena asserted. Dr. Cardenas might have a ton of degrees, she said, but when a patient needs help he just asks, "What's the problem?," without looking at them directly, then says, "Take this,'" without explaining what the medicine is for. "He is like a doctor from the Fourth Republic," Magdalena pronounced dismissively. The Fourth Republic is the forty-year period preceding the rise of the Chávez government that some celebrated as a time of stable democratic rule but others decried as a period of rising inequality.

Although I struggled to imagine Magdalena as anything other than an uncompromising politically radical health activist, she had only become interested in politics and community health work two years before I met her. In one of our interviews she described her transformation into a community health activist as a profound awakening (*un despertar*) triggered by a compassionate interaction with a Barrio Adentro doctor in 2004. Magdalena was unemployed at the time. She suffered from a painful case of rheumatoid arthritis. Then a routine office visit changed the course of her life.

> It all started because I went in for a check-up for blood pressure. I felt bad, and the doctor . . . for the first time in my life, instead of paying attention to the disease, he paid attention to me. I had been going to one doctor before, and that doctor didn't lift his face from the paper he was writing on. But this one said, "What is your life like? Do you exercise? How do you eat? What do you do every day?" He told me that I had the beginnings of hypertension, that I should exercise, not eat too many carbs, that is to say, that I should lead a healthy life. That's how [my involvement] started. I saw Lilian, the woman who was the coordinator of the Health Committee. . . . And Lilian [was outside, trying] to motivate people [to become community health workers, saying], "Look, it doesn't matter. One hour, two hours, [just] help us here with the doctor, [and] the patients, so they don't sit alone." I went up and I asked her, "How does this work? What does one have to do to do this?" I went for a blood pressure test and I ended up becoming a volunteer.

When the doctor treated Magdalena in ways that expressed care, she was caught off guard. This experience was meaningful and gratifying. It marked the beginning of her participation in a process that she claimed changed her as a person. She described Barrio Adentro as rooted in reciprocated positive affect between doctor and patient. Referring to her work with the Barrio Adentro program, she reasoned, "This vision . . . it's that as a patient I have to feel attached to what I have in order to take care of it . . . that's it. For me to love you, you have to also return to me some of what I give to you." Magdalena's job as a social promoter was to help people access health care, but she believed people wanted and deserved more than that. They wanted and deserved personable doctors who treated patients like bodies who mattered. For all these reasons, Magdalena found Dr. Cardenas inappropriate for the position of community doctor in Barrio Adentro. Overall, she said, he "doesn't want to integrate into the community."

In this cultural context, how a doctor made people feel was as important as how a doctor treated them for their medical complaints.[2] A doctor's bedside manner was never met with indifference but rather elicited pleasure or displeasure, praise or complaint. I argue that the reason for this is that for poor and working-class Venezuelans, medical encounters were not just medically but also politically significant.

Patients' narratives about doctors reveal why seemingly insignificant behaviors were so meaningful. Touch, bodily dispositions, and other communication practices were common themes in conversations with patients, who cited them as evidence of doctors' compassion and solidarity (or lack thereof). Barrio Adentro patients often distinguished between two types of doctors—good or bad—on the basis of their observations of where doctors were willing to travel to work, where they sat during consults, whether they touched patients, their tone of voice, and other embodied practices. Carolina, a middle-aged mother of two who juggled a job selling jewelry in the informal economy, taking night classes for her high school equivalency diploma, and volunteering one day a week as a Barrio Adentro community health worker, had migrated alone to Caracas at fourteen to escape a domestic employer's sexual harassment. Carolina seemed viscerally aware of the realities of social inequalities, as she revealed in an interview.

> CAROLINA: Being a humanitarian person [*una persona humanitaria*] is one of the most important parts of being a doctor.
>
> AMY: Why is it so important?
>
> CAROLINA: Because a humanitarian person attends to people with a vocation for medicine.
>
> AMY: And do you think that doctors here are humanitarian?
>
> CAROLINA: Well, those who are in the Misión [Barrio Adentro] are there because they are humanitarian. If they were not humanitarian, they would not be in the Misión.
>
> AMY: And what about the others, those who are not in Barrio Adentro? In your opinion, are they humanitarian?
>
> CAROLINA: It could be that some of them are, because I've been to private doctors and they can be, but there are others, like, I know a woman who took her little girl to a private doctor and he had an assistant who was in charge of touching the child and the assistant would tell the doctor what she found. In other words, the doctor didn't even get near the patient. What kind of a doctor is that? I couldn't believe it, but she said it's true. In the Clínica el Ávila there is a doctor like that.

In poor and working-class neighborhoods, describing a medical worker as *humanitario* was the highest praise possible. This was a person who practiced medicine as a vocation *(vocación)* and was primarily concerned for the well-being of patients. *Humanitario* was deployed in opposition to descriptors like *materialista* (materialist) and *mercantilista*. "Mercantilista" was a term with no easy English translation used to describe people who extended the capitalist logic of the marketplace to commodify something that should not be the object of commerce—in this case, health care. As patient and health activist Mariángela said, while relating how a doctor once refused to perform an emergency surgery when she could not show proof of health insurance, "Medicine demands humanity first, that you are humanitarian, but we've gotten to a point where doctors are very *mercantilistas,* they don't care about you as a person." Such criticism of doctors reflects a broader critique of market-based medicine and a strong sense of entitlement to medical services.

The substance of Carolina's criticism was that the private practice doctor sat far from a sick child and did not actually perform a physical examination. What remains implicit but essential to decode in this narrative is the socioeconomic asymmetry between Carolina's friend, likely a woman of few economic resources like Carolina, and the doctor, who worked in a well-known private clinic situated in one of the wealthiest parts of the city. It is unclear whether Carolina thought the distancing tactics she described were limited to the doctor's less wealthy clients, but she was explicit that this lack of bodily interaction was offensive and antithetical to the proper practice of medicine. Her narrative suggests that touching patients was central to being humanitarian, which she claimed was "one of the most important parts of being a doctor."

Researchers have found that specific physician behaviors, like interrupting patients, failing to acknowledge the social context of illness, and communicating disinterest in patients' suffering, can reproduce inequalities of class, gender, and race or ethnicity, among others.[3] In Latin American settings, highly bureaucratized public health services and inequalities between largely elite doctors and poor patients can render the experience of receiving (or failing to receive) medical care demeaning, disempowering, and counterproductive in terms of health outcomes.[4] In their analysis of the unequal distribution of life-giving medical services to economically and socially marginalized mothers in Brazil, Marilyn Nations and Linda-Ann Rebhun write, "Medical interactions can be seen as rituals which function to create, communicate, and direct sociopolitical realities."[5]

My observations reveal that just as some doctors' practices can reinforce socioeconomic and political marginality—like the doctor at Clínica el Ávila who would not touch the child—other types of clinical interactions can restructure social relations, activating a sense of political belonging.[6] Research participants emphasized doctor's bodily practices when they evaluated the quality and morality of individual doctors. Instances of physical intimacy between doctor and patient were interpreted as medically and morally appropriate expressions of compassion and solidarity. Embodied expressions of care and solidarity were loaded with political significance, marking patients from marginalized groups as deserving of the state's care. Andreina, who worked in the informal economy as a hairdresser out of her home before joining her husband in community organizing and health activism for the government in the early 2000s, illustrated this point.

ANDREINA: [Barrio Adentro] doctors attend to people whether they be homeless, no matter what kind of illness they have, they attend to them normally like they would with any other patient. This is very beautiful, and admirable, and the people who do this kind of work are much loved. The doctor who was here before, she would hold the homeless people, she'd change their clothes, help them, massage them. She wasn't disgusted by them, she didn't have any qualms. She said this was her job, which was very sensible, very humble. This was beautiful. She was a humanitarian person, for sure. The other doctor who's here now, she's like that too. But [Dolores, the previous doctor] was like, more spontaneous, she was more demonstrative.

AMY: And is it important for a doctor to demonstrate love?

ANDREINA: Yes.

Andreina and other people I knew valorized the notion of doctors being corporeally present and engaged with their patients and viewed compassionate touch on the part of the doctor as a sign of respect and care. That Andreina invoked the figure of the homeless person, or *indigente* (indigent), is significant. Such individuals were often portrayed as prime examples of the marginalized, excluded subject who had been abandoned by society and the state.

I observed many practices of embodied intimacy between doctors and patients in Barrio Adentro clinics, including empathic touch. If doctor and patient had met several times, they would often hug at the beginning or end of the consultation. Dr. Cardenas did not do this, which may be one of the reasons some did not think he was a good doctor. Doctora Dolores, in contrast, actually used a piece of wire to bind a chair to her desk, so patients had to sit very close to her, often brushing up against her arms and legs during consultations. She always asked patients to sit in that chair rather than against the wall or on the other side of the desk, a request that guaranteed closeness and physical intimacy during the medical encounter.

Communication practices, including eye contact, listening without interrupting, the amount of time doctors spent with patients, explanations of diagnoses and treatments, and even the use of pet names were commonly noted by patients as meaningful behaviors. Barrio Adentro medical workers routinely used an informal, intimate speech register with patients, marked by terms of endearment like *mi reina* (my queen), *mi amor* (my love), or *mi vida* (my life), reflecting a personalized and culturally normative style of talking common among kin, friends, and acquaintances.

Patients viewed personalized medical attention as evidence that doctors cared about them and respected their dignity as fellow humans. When I asked Eugenia, an elderly woman, what she thought about Barrio Adentro, she jumped at the chance to tell me: "[The Barrio Adentro doctors] have always treated me well, thanks be to God.... [T]hey look at you, they sympathize with you, [saying,] 'What's wrong? How do you feel?' And they do this with such caring, they look you in the face." In a cultural context where failing to make or maintain eye contact during conversations causes offense, patients' concerns about doctors making eye contact reflects the importance of being accorded dignity and respect in the clinic. Eugenia illustrated this point in speaking of encounters with Venezuelan doctors in a non–Barrio Adentro clinic: "Before, I went to Social Security and the doctors would sit halfway across the room." She imitated one of these doctors for me by turning her entire body and face away, assuming a harsh facial expression, and barking in a clipped voice, "¿Que tiene? ¿Que le pasa?" (What do you have? What happened to you?). After performing this interaction, she faced me and continued in her normal voice, "Can you believe that? A doctor! ... They act disgusted, like we're contagious." Her reference to "them" and "us" alluded to more than differences in professional standing: Eugenia suggested that some doctors saw the poor, people like herself, as disgusting and contagious. Indeed, an elderly woman named Teresa (mentioned in chap. 1), who was also participating in our conversation, quickly interjected with, "When you are poor ... when you are a poor person ... " Her meaning was self-evident. Teresa and Eugenia suggested that doctors' embodied distancing behaviors were rooted in class inequalities that historically structured the practice of medicine and served to reinforce patients' marginalized status.

Eugenia's statements were representative of many comments I heard from people who used Barrio Adentro services. For these patients, the technical competence of doctors was important and usually assumed. However, Barrio

Adentro patients focused not on the doctors' technical competence but on the way they made them feel about their social and class position. Patients criticized doctors when their behaviors emphasized status asymmetries.

A DIFFERENT MODEL OF BIOMEDICINE

Listening to Barrio Adentro patients, I learned that when people responded with pleasure to encounters with doctors, they were responding to doctors who were acting on a distinct biomedical epistemology. This form of medicine borrows from Cuba's biopsychosocial model of health, which posits that sickness cannot be understood outside of the social context in which it emerges. This medical model recognizes that disorder in people's social and economic lives can lead to bodily ailments. Bodily ailments may thus express social, political, and economic distress. Doctors socialized into a biopsychosocial model of health often learn a style of patient interaction that emphasizes attending to the whole person and their social context rather than simply focusing on a biophysical pathology. This is what Magdalena was referring to when she said, "For the first time in my life, instead of paying attention to the disease, [the doctor] paid attention to *me*." The Barrio Adentro doctor who treated Madgalena refocused their interaction from her presenting complaint (blood pressure) to an assessment of her overall well-being. In Barrio Adentro this holistic approach is termed *medicina integral,* or integrated (or comprehensive) medicine.

The philosophy and epistemology of Cuban medicine reflected a culturally specific form of biomedicine that dovetailed with Chávez's promises to end neoliberal policies and promote social justice. Since the 1960s the Cuban government has championed the idea of medicine as a basic right. Doctors are portrayed as activists, as living embodiments of socialist sacrifice and solidarity who practice medicine as a vocation, not as a commercial enterprise.[7] The epistemology of Cuban medicine emphasized not just the social and psychological context of health and illness (the biopsychosocial approach) but also providing medical care in the neighborhoods where patients live and cultivating personalized doctor-patient relationships.[8] This approach resonates more broadly with the regional social justice movement known as Latin American social medicine (LASM).[9] The sociologist Christina Perez's three-year ethnographic study of community medicine in Cuba led her to conclude, "The doctor and nurse role in Cuba is very different from the 'medical professional' in modern biomedicine.... In the family doctor *consultorio* [clinic] humanity is a methodology; it is part of the practice of community based medicine. It does not happen by chance, but is part of the doctor's training."[10]

The political and humanistic values shaping Cuban medical practice informed the pedagogy and clinical practice of Barrio Adentro workers and students. Barrio Adentro medical students I met expressed pride in working in a socialized health system. A medical student in Santa Teresa named Yolanda told me that anyone training to become a Barrio Adentro doctor "has a future as a human, not as a materialist."

My research revealed that patients read a lot of meaning into doctors' embodied practices (i.e., what doctors did with their bodies in clinical encounters). For example, Magdalena suggested that a doctor's lack of eye contact demonstrated a poor bedside manner and disregard for her well-being. Thinking about the doctor's gaze is useful for understanding the way that different epistemologies of biomedicine can produce different clinical habits in doctors. Depending on patients' expectations and desires, these clinical habits can elicit pleasure and a sense of solidarity or displeasure and a sense of dehumanization.

In his history of biomedicine Michel Foucault theorized about the medical gaze, a way of seeing specific to Western biomedicine.[11] The medical gaze refers to doctors' habit of focusing on particular body parts, diseases, and pathogens to understand problems of biological functioning. This laser-focused visualization has resulted in medical breakthroughs, but critics say it comes at a cost because the medical gaze can dehumanize patients. The anthropologist Beverly Davenport explains the medical gaze as "seeing a 'case' or a 'condition' rather than a human being."[12] Attempting to isolate and objectify pathology in the body gives doctors an opportunity to ignore the person standing in front of them. Biomedicine thus runs the risk of becoming depersonalized to the point that some doctors might diagnose and treat a disease without ever looking a patient in the eyes or talking to them about their complaints. The kind of medicine that Barrio Adentro promised and the kind of medicine that patients desired did not rely on the medical gaze for efficacy. Looking patients in the eyes reflected a medical commitment to recognizing the whole person as a product of their social context. Patients also interpreted it as politically relevant. Patients took pleasure in doctors looking them in the eyes because they interpreted this behavior as identifying them as a person worthy of respect.

We know from other anthropologists' work that cultural dispositions and values come to be embodied in medical training through processes of socialization and are later expressed in doctors' engagements with patients.[13] For example, students in some medical programs may learn to sit, speak, and listen in ways that reflect their political commitment to acknowledging and responding to the socioeconomic disempowerment of their patients.[14] In her research on Bolivian medical students training in the Cuban medical system, Alyssa Bernstein described how a Cuban doctor urged a Bolivian medical student to stop rushing through consultations and to "sit and listen, and listen to everything that the patient has to say," after which one patient announced that just talking about her problems with the medical student helped her pain go away.[15] Bernstein also found that Bolivian students training under Cuban doctors were explicitly taught the importance of laughing, joking, and smiling to ease patients' worries and minimize the hierarchy of the doctor-patient encounter.[16] In a Barrio Adentro clinic I observed a Cuban doctor interrupt her medical students while they practiced clinical interviewing. A student asked another student, who was playing the role of patient, "What are your symptoms?" The doctor stopped the role-playing scenario, saying, "Don't ask about the patient's *symptoms*. That's a technical term; they might not know it. Ask them instead, 'What's wrong?,' 'Why did you come to see me today?,' or 'What kind of problem are you having?,' and let them tell you in their own words." In this teaching moment, the doctor encouraged her medical students to rethink verbal norms of clinical interaction to appear more personable and easier to understand.

Patients responded with pleasure to affectively charged medical interactions that they believed expressed love and compassion. Many Barrio Adentro patients noted sensory details like doctors' speech, mannerisms, and physical contact with them and, using existing cultural logics, interpreted these embodied practices as having aesthetic, moral, and political meanings.[17] Their responses were informed by regionally specific desires for personalized medicine. In Venezuela, the fame and valorization of the "doctor of the poor" José Gregorio informed normative models of medicine, including expectations that doctors practice medicine as a vocation, be easily accessible to patients of all social classes, and treat patients in the neighborhoods where they live.

Local and regional desires for personalized medicine likely influenced how officials presented Barrio Adentro. The Chávez government cultivated expectations for a "loving biomedicine" through publicity and other media.

One example was a glossy booklet published by the Barrio Adentro head office for public distribution. The cover shows a photo of a pretty female doctor gently examining a sleeping baby in the dim light of a makeshift barrio clinic. Curvilinear graphics and flowers surrounded the photo and the booklet's title, *Barrio Adentro: Una obra de corazón* (literally, "A Work of the Heart").[18] Graphic designers replaced the letter "o" in the word *corazón* with a plump red heart to impress on readers that the health program offered love in addition to medical services.

It was not just in its health services that the revolutionary government marketed itself as a source of love and compassion for the people. Slogans like "Love is the motor of the revolution" (Amor es el motor de la revolucíon) showed up on government publicity across the city. Chávez appeared on television or in posters hugging and serenading members of the public, embodying a warm, protective persona. One government poster featured a photograph of Chávez hugging an elderly Afro-Venezuelan woman, with the buoyant slogan, "¡Que siga la emoción!," roughly translated as "Keeping spirits high!" The entire wall of the waiting room of one Barrio Adentro clinic I visited was taken up by a mural depicting Chávez holding a puppy in the center of a bright green field while a beaming pair of children stood beside him.

Although government media seemed to promise intimacy, love, and compassion to the people at every turn, in practice the most likely means of experiencing something akin to love or care from the government was in the hands of a medical worker (although, of course, not all of them actually communicated love or care). Other government programs lacked the same opportunities for intimate encounters with government workers who listened, touched, and cared for people. Inside the clinic the national ideology of love and compassion for the poor could take tangible form. For most people, doctors were the closest approximation of a physical instantiation of the government touching them, recognizing them, and expressing care for them.

WHAT DOCTORS SYMBOLIZED

When I first began hearing narratives of clinical interactions, I was surprised by the emotion that people expressed when talking about going to the doctor. They seemed so happy. They really seemed to enjoy visiting the doctor's office. I even observed patients speaking with excitement about seeing the dentist for cleanings, teeth extractions, and dentures. To my North American ears this all sounded strange, probably because in the United States doctors' visits are not eagerly anticipated and enjoyed but rather often dreaded and avoided. Comedians in the United States poke fun at the doctor-patient encounter as something inherently awkward and disempowering for patients: having to sit in the waiting room, having to wear those flimsy gowns, and so on. I was skeptical of the glowing reports people gave of their experiences with new government clinics. However, I learned that for poor and working-class Venezuelans, going to the doctor means something very different from what it means to most Americans.

My observations revealed a politics of interaction between doctors and patients inside the clinics. People weren't simply gaining access to free diagnoses and treatments; they also felt they were engaging in politically meaningful relationships with doctors.

A consistent pattern in my interlocutors' discourse was the dichotomization of Barrio Adentro doctors and non–Barrio Adentro doctors. Zoraida's commentary below reflects the way many patients talked about the two types of doctors, as if they were from different worlds. Zoraida was different from many patients I interviewed, because she was a middle-class professional living in a wealthy neighborhood in Caracas. However, her commentary exemplifies the comparisons I recorded in my field notes time and again.

> Personally, I have received extraordinary care from the Cuban doctors . . . the times that I've gone—they've been for very small matters, like I had a sore throat or something—I've always received extraordinary attention.
>
> They have a totally different philosophy than our doctors. Our doctors are arrogant, materialists. They charge you for consultations that, one woman from the barrio, she had to work a month to get the money together.
>
> They make you wait. What do you think about this: you have to wait five hours in a doctor's office and the nurse comes out and tells you: "The doctor is not coming in today," and you're dying, you know? . . .
>
> One goes to Barrio Adentro and the *doctora* or *doctor,* they're always there for you, they give you the best they can give, they provide good treatment, they chat with you, listen to you . . . because they have a philosophy of life that's different from ours. Sometimes you go to a doctor here, and he won't even look you in the face.

The qualities Zoraida attributed to "our doctors"—arrogance, materialism, disinterest in patients' suffering—are at odds with the qualities she attributes to the "Cuban doctors." Cuban doctors were conflated with Barrio Adentro doctors here as they were in many other patients' conversations, even though about 20 percent of all Barrio Adentro doctors were Venezuelan at the time I conducted this research.[19] Zoraida explained the differences as stemming from different "philosophies of life"—likely a reference to Cuban socialism and the philosophy of Cuban medicine.

Viki, the nursing student, also revealed her understanding of Cuban doctors as qualitatively different from Venezuelan doctors. For her, bodily practices such as whether doctors wore their white coats revealed their attitudes toward patients.

> You don't see this pretentiousness in the Cuban doctors in Barrio Adentro, they are very simple people; you have to ask them if they are doctors because they're not constantly wearing their white coats. They have their white coats, but when they leave, they take them off. . . . They don't have this . . . pretension, you see. They don't look down on everybody else. Instead, everyone is equal.

For Viki, a doctor who wears a white coat when not on duty, when there is no pragmatic reason for doing so, is inscribing status differences on his or her body that should be downplayed, not highlighted. She classifies Cuban Barrio Adentro doctors as egalitarian and Venezuelan, non–Barrio Adentro doctors as elitist on the basis of doctors' bodily habitus.

At the same time, people acknowledged that treating patients holistically and with respect was not a new concept in Venezuela. Medical workers noted that the positive qualities of medicine associated with Barrio Adentro historically informed Venezuelan medical practice (recall the beloved Dr. José Gregorio) and were inculcated in their medical training prior to Barrio Adentro but that in the past few decades positive values in clinical medicine had been overshadowed by negative values like materialism and a disregard for poor patients. For example, the Barrio Adentro nurse Alejandra (whose husband was a private practice doctor) told me:

> In the Military Hospital where I [previously] worked, as well as in the private clinics, . . . the humanitarian component has been lost. One works primarily to earn money, without paying attention to a patient's mood or to how a patient is feeling.
>
> In community work [Barrio Adentro], in contrast, it's like we say, the flip side of the tortilla. Why? Because, you see, here you feel the humanity more. You listen to the patient, you listen to his or her problems. In other words, you

practically become a psychologist for these patients. Here, there are no class distinctions. Here in Barrio Adentro a patient may come in who's able to pay for a private clinic, all the way down to an indigent who doesn't even have the money to pay for his own bandages in a hospital.

For Alejandra, the main difference between Barrio Adentro work and medical practice in other settings was not the nationality of its workers but "the humanitarian component" embedded in the political orientation to "community work." She clarified the meaning of the term "humanitario" by locating it in compassionate face-to-face interactions ("You listen to the patient . . . you practically become [their] psychologist") and in the willingness of the clinic and its staff to care for all people, regardless of their ability to pay. For Alejandra, despite various problems that patients and medical workers freely acknowledged (unreliable supplies of medications, problems filling vacant posts, low pay for workers), Barrio Adentro represented a valorized alternative to the supposedly normalized practice of Venezuelan medicine, which was seen to involve "earning money without paying attention . . . to how a patient is feeling."

People working in and using Barrio Adentro clinics viewed the doctors in these clinics as literally embodying different values and thus engaging in different kinds of doctor-patient exchanges from those of doctors working outside the Barrio Adentro system (although when pressed, patients acknowledged that reality was more complex than this opposition suggested). The dichotomy between "good" Barrio Adentro doctors and "bad" non–Barrio Adentro doctors was stark and politicized, suggesting that this opposition was symbolically evocative for patients.

In fact, different forms of medical embodiment represented different moral economies of medicine and different political systems. Barrio Adentro doctors were emblematic of a model of medicine that challenged the inequities associated with market-based medical systems. These doctors represented the leftist Chávez government, which promised to redistribute national wealth and challenge social and political exclusions. Descriptions of non–Barrio Adentro doctors evoked market-based medicine and the neoliberal governments that came before Chávez. This dichotomy made doctor-patient interactions politically charged experiences with implications for how patients understood their position in the sociopolitical order.

The negative values patients often read in non–Barrio Adentro doctors' behaviors were the same *anti-valores,* or anti-values, that patients (and state officials) associated with neoliberalism as a cultural logic, including individualism, materialism, and profit-driven medicine. In contrast, the positive values patients often attributed to Barrio Adentro doctors, like solidarity, egalitarianism, and humanitarianism, mapped onto values they associated with an idealized Venezuelan past, the Chávez government (including Chávez himself), and an idealized Venezuelan future. In the dichotomy patients presented of good and bad doctors, memories of state austerity measures and state abandonment became personalized in the caricature of the uncaring, materialist Venezuelan doctor, while the idealized Barrio Adentro doctor represented contemporary state institutions fulfilling the state's responsibility to care for citizens. Of course, these memories were context-dependent and were made and remade through interactions with others, often as a response to present-day concerns and struggles.[20] The polarization of Venezuelan society along class and political lines shaped how people remembered past governments, evaluated state policies, and interpreted the bodily practices of doctors in different biomedical settings. Stark, dichotomous representations of the different forms of medical practice thought to characterize Barrio Adento and non–Barrio Adentro doctors communicated patients' feelings of inclusion or exclusion at the level of nation-state belonging.[21]

Because doctors' encounters symbolized different approaches to medicine and different political legacies in Venezuela, medical care could instantiate for patients a sense of sociopolitical marginality or a sense of sociopolitical belonging (fig. 9). For patients of Barrio Adentro, doctor-patient interactions could be experienced as disempowering or empowering, depending on how patients read doctors' embodied dispositions, values, and practices during the consultation. Encounters with disinterested, condescending doctors could reinforce patients' sense of social, political, and economic marginalization, while experiences of intimate, compassionate doctor-patient interactions could signify a righting of historical wrongs on the part of the revolutionary state and mark patients' deservingness.

Given that Cuban doctors in Venezuela belonged to the Cuban government's internationalist medical aid missions, one might wonder whether my Venezuelan research participants viewed their presence as a form of transnational solidarity. They did, to some extent. Venezuelans knew of Cuba's reputation for sending medical workers abroad to help marginalized people. They often described Cuban doctors as *solidarios,* a term that translates as "supportive of/in solidarity with/standing up" for others out of a sense of empa-

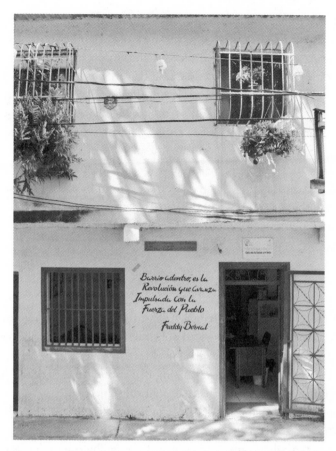

FIGURE 9. Barrio Adentro neighborhood clinic operating out of a home. Quotation from then-mayor of Libertador Municipality reads, "Barrio Adentro is the revolution that advances with the strength of the people." Photo by the author.

thy and care. Research participants explained that Cuban doctors were this way because of (a) medical training that emphasized empathy with patients and understanding their social conditions; (b) socialist upbringing that prepared them to be collectivist, egalitarian members of society; and (c) the material difficulties of life in Cuba that helped them understand what it was like to live in a poor or working-class neighborhood in Venezuela.

At the same time, Venezuelan research participants viewed Cubans' presence in Venezuela as not solely or even primarily an expression of transnational solidarity but rather an instantiation of the Venezuelan government caring for its people and fulfilling a constitutional mandate to provide health care. Cuba's medical work in Venezuela was unlike other missions abroad both in scale and in the fact that the Venezuelan government paid for medical aid with oil—one hundred thousand barrels a day. The Cuban government could not have sent so many of its medical workers (approximately one in five of all doctors in Cuba left to work in Barrio Adentro) without the incentives provided by Venezuela. While the arrangement was an example of transnational solidarity and individual Cubans were viewed as working in solidarity with their Venezuelan patients, in the minds of Venezuelan research participants the Cuban doctors worked in Barrio Adentro because of the empathy and solidarity of the Venezuelan government, especially their president, Hugo Chávez.

THE PLEASURE OF INCLUSION

One of the explicit aims of Barrio Adentro was to integrate marginalized individuals into the realm of valued political subjects by giving them a range of services that provided immediate medical assistance and in doing so, fulfilled a long-standing promise of patrimonial entitlements to the nation's oil wealth. But my research reveals that political subjectivities were not transformed merely by expanding access to medical services. Central to the political processes at play in the provision of state health care were the intimate aspects of medical encounters. Because of the symbolism of doctors in this context, how the doctor interacted with patients in face-to-face encounters were shot through with political significance. Just as interacting with a "mercantilista" doctor could reinforce patients' sociopolitical marginality, interacting with a "humanitarian" doctor could instantiate a sense of sociopolitical belonging. The importance of the doctor's body is historically and culturally contingent, dependent on local conventions and expectations in the realms of medicine and the state. It is something that we should pay attention to when studying people's experiences of health care in other cultural settings.

These findings are unusual in that they demonstrate how a sense of belonging and empowerment can result from poor people's interactions with government doctors. We know from anthropological research that doctor-patient interactions can be sites of political negotiation and contestation, often serving as microcosms of large-scale social, political, and economic relationships. But research usually shows clinical interactions having a negative effect on poor and otherwise marginalized patients by reproducing their unequal status or further marginalizing them. The idea that medical interactions reinforce social inequalities has been so well supported by ethnographic research that it would be easy to assume that medical interactions inevitably reproduce patients' marginalized status.

Not all research suggests that clinical interactions reinforce power inequalities.[22] In some cases anthropologists have shown that medical interactions may empower patients in social, economic, and political hierarchies.[23] In Ecuador, Elizabeth Roberts found that lower- and middle-class research participants valorized intimate interactions with private practice doctors and sought out personalized relationships with these doctors, who "greeted patients with kisses and endearments."[24] In this case establishing relationships with private practice doctors was empowering because accessing the kind of medical care associated with elite and wealthy Ecuadorians indexed upward social mobility in a rigid class hierarchy. In contrast, Barrio Adentro patients valorized intimate doctor-patient interactions in the context of government health care, where such interactions produced a sense of radical political transformation. For Venezuelan research participants, compassionate medical treatment evidenced rising equality across social classes and more responsive state institutions.

Venezuelan patients who had long resented what they saw as the state's failure to follow through on promises to use national oil wealth to provide for its citizens came to see the state's efforts to address sociopolitical inequalities in the dispositions of its medical workers. In clinical interactions, patients sought not just medical goods and services but also expressions of recognition, respect, care, and solidarity from these state agents. Regional moral economies of medicine shaped poor patients' expectations that doctors comport themselves in ways that validated patients' dignity and worth. In addition, Barrio Adentro patients expected concordance between what was promised in state discourse (demarginalization, collective sharing of oil wealth) and what was provided in doctor-patient interactions. Caring treatment signaled their improved position vis-à-vis the government and Venezuelan society and as such served as a source of pleasure for patients.

During this period the government instituted many social programs intended to improve people's material conditions and reverse a history of social inequalities. Unique among these programs, Barrio Adentro enabled close, personal interactions with people who worked for and symbolically represented the Chávez government. Going to the doctor was a special opportunity to literally feel like a body who mattered to the state. Clinical intimacies were meaningful because they enacted large-scale political dynamics, either reproducing or reshaping macropolitical relationships between poor and working-class people, the government, and Venezuelan society.

FOUR

Beyond Biomedicine

A VISITOR TO SANTA TERESA COULD NOT HELP but notice the neighborhood's spiritual healing and plant-based medicine shops, especially along the main shopping street, Avenida Baralt. They were too numerous and too lively to ignore. Tinctures and figurines stood at attention in neat rows, their rainbow hues beckoning to passersby. Herb and plant bundles spilled onto the sidewalks as if the shop's architecture could not contain their healing potential. These shops reflected residents' enthusiasm for different forms of popular medicine—medical traditions that derived their authority from people rather than from an external authority like the state or the scientific elite.[1] Research participants drew no hard-and-fast boundaries between biomedicine and other medical systems, alternating between approaches and combining them as they saw fit. When government services like Barrio Adentro moved inside neighborhoods they joined diverse medical traditions already enjoying a wide following.

Regardless of their excitement about Barrio Adentro, poor and working-class Caraqueños did not view the program as replacing popular health practices such as spiritual healing, herbal remedies, or acupuncture. This finding should not surprise us. Medical pluralism—the proliferation of multiple, seemingly competing medical systems—has been the norm in state societies throughout history.[2] When biomedically oriented programs like Barrio Adentro enter new social spaces they tend to operate alongside existing medical traditions in a plural medical landscape.

What is surprising is that as Barrio Adentro expanded biomedical services in poor neighborhoods, the Bolivarian government changed how people experienced medical pluralism in unexpected ways. By celebrating the integrity of popular medical traditions (historically associated with marginalized

Venezuelans) while radically expanding access to biomedicine (historically associated with elites), officials disrupted hierarchies of status and access that differentiated biomedicine from other healing traditions. Investing popular medicine with greater prestige and authority contributed to a broader sociopolitical shift toward greater equality for marginalized people. Venezuelans took pleasure navigating a medically plural landscape that symbolized greater empowerment and inclusion.

POWER RELATIONS AND MEDICAL PLURALISM

"Medical pluralism" does not refer to a value-neutral medical marketplace unaffected by power relations. Rather, it tends to reflect and reinforce social hierarchies.[3] In complex state societies, medical systems come to be associated with the social classes, genders, and racial or ethnic groups that constitute their base of patients and practitioners. Medical systems accrue different levels of prestige and authority that map onto broader social inequalities.[4] Some forms of medicine become more powerful institutionally and economically, limiting access to less privileged social groups.

Biomedicine has enjoyed an especially powerful position vis-à-vis other medical systems since gaining legitimacy across Europe and the Americas in the late 1800s.[5] Some people assume biomedicine's rise to prominence was inevitable because its scientific basis gave practitioners an advantage in curing disease, but this is not the full story; political factors played a role as well. Proponents of biomedicine fought hard to position it as the exclusive authority on medicine, often seeking to delegitimize other medical systems in the process.[6] The anthropologist and physician Arthur Kleinman argues that biomedicine is unique among healing systems in being "monotheistic," meaning that its practitioners see it as the only authentic form of medicine and express intolerance for other medical traditions.[7] This monotheism explains why proponents invested such effort to position it as the dominant medical system. Historians of medicine in Latin America recount a long history of biomedical experts working with state officials to enshrine biomedicine as economically and institutionally dominant over other healing traditions, for example, by creating licensing procedures to authorize only biomedical practitioners to practice medicine. In Latin America biomedical doctors often became politicians and shaped government policies.[8] In Latin America and elsewhere, biomedicine's supporters framed its practices as modern, scientific, and therapeutically superior to other medical systems.

Biomedical dominance was never totalizing—people worldwide have continued to practice and use popular medicine—but efforts to delegitimize nonbiomedical practices introduced stereotypes of popular medical traditions as backward, irrational, and ineffective. Negative stereotypes similarly accrued to the people most strongly identified with popular medical traditions. In Latin America this usually meant poor people, women, and indigenous people and other people of color. Efforts to economically and institutionally subordinate popular medicine to biomedicine reinforced class, gender, and ethnic or racial inequalities in society. Even socialist governments (including Cuba and the USSR) unintentionally stigmatized marginalized social groups by making biomedicine the official healing system and prohibiting others in order to "modernize" society and promote scientific thinking among the people.[9]

Venezuelan officials under Chávez did not follow the historical pattern of delegitimizing popular medical traditions to promote adherence to new biomedical services. Instead the government disrupted biomedicine's authority in subtle (sometimes unintentional) ways and intentionally acknowledged the value of popular medical traditions. As a result, poor and working-class Caraqueños maintained a great deal of control over how they sought health care. While people experienced increased choice in biomedical care, better access to biomedicine did not cost people their dignity or prevent access to popular medicine. By respecting and legitimizing medical traditions associated with historically disempowered groups, the government respected and legitimized members of these groups as well. All of this served as a source of pleasure for people. In the sections that follow I explain how this process played out from research participants' point of view. I begin with two case studies showing how individuals experienced medical pluralism under Chávez's leadership.

Nilda and Her Parents

Nilda was a sixty-year-old Afro-Venezuelan woman who loved Barrio Adentro but distrusted biomedicine. I met her when she visited Doctora Mercedes in the Barrio Adentro clinic. Tall and well dressed and with a bubbly personality, Nilda swept Mercedes into a big hug as she entered the room and confirmed that Mercedes would drop by her house for a visit after work.

They settled into talking about current events, drawing me into a rapid-fire conversation about global affairs. Nilda praised Raul Castro's upcoming visit to Brazil because it would make Cuba less isolated. She and Mercedes spoke admiringly about Barack Obama, who had just won the 2008 presidential election in the United States. They agreed he had "spark" and intelligence and would greatly benefit the country. Nilda informed Mercedes that she had been going to acupuncture and taking the medication Mercedes gave her. It took care of her infection, but she still had neck pain. Mercedes offered a box of naproxen to treat the pain and inflammation.

When talking to me that day, Nilda enumerated how she benefited from Barrio Adentro and referred to the *cambio grande* (big change) that had been happening in Venezuela since Chávez took office. Nilda seemed more financially comfortable than other Barrio Adentro patients I met. One of her sons lived in San Diego (through whom she acquired a green card), and she visited him every three months. When I visited her home for a formal interview, I found that she lived at the western edge of Santa Teresa, across the street from the RCTV cable network that made global headlines after losing its free broadcast license over its purported role in the 2002 coup against Chávez. Nilda shared a large apartment with her mother, who was in her eighties, and her father, who was ninety-six. She included her mother in our interview, which took place in their living room with the public television station Canal 8 running in the background. She also invited her housekeeper to discuss her experience bringing her son to weekly speech therapy at Barrio Adentro.

Nilda commented that their preference for Barrio Adentro and for specific doctors meant they went out of their way to go to certain clinics even if others were more conveniently located. Nilda joked, "We stalk Dolores. Hahaha! [Now she is] in San Bernadino. We went there recently, I took my mom, and then I took four of her other patients." Doctora Dolores used to work in Santa Teresa but was reassigned to a Barrio Adentro clinic in a different neighborhood. Nilda and her parents continued to seek her out, though Nilda also befriended Doctora Mercedes, who replaced her.

One reason they preferred Barrio Adentro doctors had to do with the belief that they provided better outcomes with less medical intervention. Nilda's mother and father previously used private clinics with health insurance from their former employers (the Post Office and the Ministry of Communications, respectively). But as Nilda's mother said of the private clinic, "Instead of getting better, all we did was get sicker. They gave us a lot of antibiotics, and things like that, you see? . . . Afterwards, I told Nilda that I didn't want her to take me there again." Nilda explained that the private clinic mismanaged her parents' pharmaceutical regimes.

> My dad fell. And, emotionally, I imagine that things started to pile up, his blood pressure was irregular. So I took him to the [private] clinic, and it was worse for him there, with pills here, there, and everywhere. Then Dolores came along, and she told him that the medicine that he was going to take was a vitamin. He needed something to decrease his cholesterol and nothing else. And then he stopped taking the pills for his blood pressure, all that poison the [private] clinic was giving him. . . . It's a business, love. The laboratories pay the doctors, or better yet, doctors benefit from prescribing those expensive medicines.

Nilda complained that prescription medications were not only costly for patients; they could be unnecessary and even harmful ("poison" in her terms). Her family felt that the fewer pharmaceuticals needed, the better. They praised the physical therapists at Barrio Adentro for making weekly visits to their home for the past few months, citing this as having a major impact on persistent health problems each was experiencing. All three attended dance therapy led by the Cuban trainer Darwin at the school near their house. Nilda and her mother also visited a homeopath-acupuncturist regularly, paying 250 Bs (approximately US$116) per consultation. In addition, they had been visiting an acupuncture school every week for the past two years for reduced cost sessions (15 Bs / US$7 per visit). They knew they could access acupuncture for free through a Barrio Adentro rehabilitation center but thought it better to let "people that need it more" take advantage of the government-provided free treatments. In addition to visiting popular medicine specialists, Nilda's family relied on plant-based home remedies (including teas and infusions) to treat common health complaints.

She believed popular medicine was not merely an alternative to biomedical care, but could cure the damage done by biomedicine gone awry. Nilda had battled an addiction to lexotanil (also known as bromazepam), a prescription anti-anxiety drug similar to valium. She used acupuncture and homeopathy to overcome her addiction and said she continued to use acupuncture now to "balance herself." Nilda explained, "Many times pharmaceutical medicine cures one thing and hurts another, see? And so much medicine makes you sick, girl. So you look for alternatives."

Nilda's distrust of private practice biomedical doctors led her to avoid private medical care and embrace Barrio Adentro. She said Venezuelan private practice doctors overprescribed medications because they cared more about profit than about their patients' health. Although Nilda did not explain how doctors profited from prescriptions, other research participants explained that unscrupulous doctors sent patients to specific pharmacies to buy medication and received a payoff in return. She and her mother commented on other aspects of corruption in the Venezuelan medical system that made them view doctors in private clinics with suspicion. Many doctors worked simultaneously in private practice and public hospitals, and research participants like Nilda thought it was common knowledge that doctors stole government-provided equipment and medications from the hospitals where they worked to stock their private clinics. Corrupt and profit-oriented doctors led Nilda's family to forgo their private health insurance benefits (which, ironically, they received as a government benefit for having worked in the civil service) after Barrio Adentro arrived. Like other research participants, they viewed Barrio Adentro as relatively immune from corruption because it operated as a separate public health system with its own administrators, distribution networks, and training practices, not to mention the fact that Cuban health workers were widely viewed as incorruptible.

When they did seek biomedicine, Nilda's family preferred Barrio Adentro over long-established public hospitals because they could access Barrio Adentro care much more quickly. Her mother compared a recent visit to a Barrio Adentro diagnostic center where she received an echocardiogram and X-ray "immediately, immediately, we weren't even there two hours," to a visit Nilda's father made to a hospital emergency room where he arrived in the morning and wasn't taken into intensive care until 10:00 P.M. Nilda explained, "You know that whatever ache or pain you have you can run over to Barrio Adentro. I do it." Nilda's family took comfort in Barrio Adentro's convenience and quality of care.

Even though Nilda's family had private insurance and could access private health care, they clearly preferred Barrio Adentro. This might surprise those who assume that regardless of cultural context, government health care is substandard and stigmatized compared to private medicine. But this was not the case for many people, including Nilda, who believed private clinics offered no advantage over government clinics. In fact, the anecdotes Nilda provided of her family's experiences suggested that she believed private biomedicine was the riskiest choice for medical care. This was most apparent in her story of medical malpractice by a gynecologist.

> I used to go to a private doctor, to a gynecologist. [Once,] he put the instrument in, it broke, and he took the instrument out. He *said* he took it out. It turns out that after I started going to Barrio Adentro, I arranged for them to do a routine gynecological exam and they found a severe infection of the cervix. They sent me to where there is a . . . military fortress, something like that [Hospital Militar, a government hospital now open to the public], where there are Cuban doctors. And they did an ultrasound, and they found out that half of the instrument was still inside of me. It was embedded in my uterus. . . . That happened to me with a private doctor. And who took it out for me? Barrio Adentro saw it, and they sent me to the Military Hospital and they took it out there.

Nilda's mother told her to show me the ultrasound revealing the embedded instrument, but Nilda shuddered and said she threw the image away. She did not want a physical reminder of the experience. In spite of their distress, the family never denounced the doctor because he became a high-ranking administrator in one of the medical schools and he was "half related" to them because he married into the family of Nilda's parents' friends.

Nilda and her mother had plenty of choices for biomedical care but often favored popular medical practices, which they perceived as less harmful, even when these treatments cost more than a biomedical treatment. These enthusiastic supporters of Barrio Adentro used its services selectively, incorporating them into a health regimen that gave equal or greater weight to alternative healing methods.

Andreina

Andreina was a fifty-four-year-old naturalized Venezuelan of mestiza origin. I got to know her through a course for community health workers in Santa Teresa. Short and sturdy with a no-nonsense attitude, Andreina was originally from Colombia but had been living in Caracas all of her adult life. In an interview I conducted after one of our classes, Andreina explained the importance of health care in Chávez's Venezuela. Spending time in Colombia gave her insight into the significance of Barrio Adentro. She said:

> When I was in Colombia recently, about three or four years ago, I went to the doctor because my daughter got sick, and in Colombia if you don't have

money to buy medicine or you don't have money so they will see you, you die. That was something over there that I didn't like at all. And I said to myself, "How different from Venezuela." In Venezuela you go to the Cuban doctor's clinic and . . . you don't have to buy anything at all. In Colombia . . . everything is really expensive. I don't know how the poor people live over there.

Andreina was grateful that Barrio Adentro offered straightforward visits in which patients got what they needed without administrative hurdles or fees. Andreina appreciated that Barrio Adentro let patients choose which clinics to visit. For Andreina and others, this freedom of choice lent a sense of excess to the availability of government health care that offered its own kind of satisfaction.

> In one barrio or parish there are two or three clinics, and you can choose the one that you want to go to, they are public and they take you. Here [Santa Teresa] there are various clinics, for example, and in San Juan there are quite a few. If I want to go to San Juan because it is close by for me, I'll go to San Juan, and if I want to go to Santa Teresa, I'll go to that one.

Research participants remarked on the number of government clinics they could visit whenever they wanted. They could visit one walk-in clinic on Monday and a different walk-in clinic the following day, without any questions from staff or administrators (even though doing so might have impeded their continuity of care). With the exception of Barrio Adentro's rehabilitation clinics, where patients followed a schedule of visits for weeks or months, all clinics were ambulatory (walk-in) services requiring no appointments for same-day attention. Although most people felt no need to try many clinics and stayed with one or two clinics they favored, this sense of abundance and freedom produced a kind of pleasure for people like Andreina who knew what it felt like to lack access to health care.[10]

Andreina and her husband worked as community health workers. She spent hours working with individuals to prepare informes, documents requesting government assistance for a medical need that could not be met by government clinics, usually things like wheelchairs, canes, operations. Andreina delivered informes to different offices: the mayor's office of Libertador Municipality, the Fondo Único Social (an office created by the Chávez government that funded citizens' requests for social development, health, and education), and Miraflores (the presidential palace). Andreina explained:

There are *so many* institutions that give out aid to the people [*el pueblo*], to the community, to the parishes. A lot of institutions, and between all of those is the PDVSA [state oil company] that helps people, with regard to health and everything else.... [For serious health problems] we point the majority of people to Miraflores, they fix the problem for them quickly there....

I have been present to see a lot of people who needed operations that cost 20 or 30 million [Bs] [approximately US$9,300–$14,000]. I have seen them give a check to the person to cover all the expenses of the operation and of the clinic where they are going to have the operation done.

The Fondo Único Social and Miraflores filled some of the gaps in specialized medical care that have long plagued the fractured public health system. Andreina noted that now people could petition the government to pay for treatments that public hospitals could not provide, whereas before treatments in private clinics were usually limited to people who could pay out of pocket.

This piecemeal solution was less than ideal. It required considerable effort to coordinate a request and verify medical need, which was why health promoters like Andreina helped patients navigate the process. Yet I observed many people praising this arrangement and very few deriding it. The ad hoc system of intervention seemed to support popular perceptions that a surfeit of government agencies provided medical assistance.

Many people suggested that seeking help in this way was good because it made people more active agents in promoting their own health. As Andreina said:

There are a lot of people who are working as volunteers, a lot, because they want to help the people and they want this process and they want to move forward.... You don't see as much poverty now because the people know and they go looking for assistance, they are moving forward of their own volition and you guide them too to resolve their problems, whether that be a housing, health, or economic problem.

Although Andreina praised the new ways to access biomedicine, she was not a person whom anthropologists would describe as a biomedicalized subject. When it came to her own health and that of her daughter, who had Down's syndrome, Andreina hesitated to adopt biomedical solutions. For example, she refused government assistance for a surgery to improve her daughter's airway obstruction and speech problems. After careful consideration Andreina treated her daughter with natural medicines, even though Chávez personally took an interest in her daughter's medical care. Andreina explained:

The last time I was close to [Chávez] ... I was in Maracay [to watch a sports event]. He passed by where we were waiting for him, saw my daughter, and told me, "This little girl needs help." He said, "Help her for me, write down her name for me," and right away one of his assistants came back to take down my information and all of that to help my daughter.

They called me many times to have me bring in the papers, but I didn't bring them in. It hurt me a lot, but, well, it happened for a reason. Maybe God didn't want my daughter to be operated on, maybe it was going to bring me trouble or something.

Andreina worried that if her daughter's tonsils were removed she might face problems later due to a weakened immune system. Andreina preferred "to give her natural treatment, home remedies." She collected remedies from friends who were doctors as well as from naturopaths she met. She used home remedies herself for problems like dizzy spells that had been bothering her. For her daughter she preferred to leave things in God's hands "until he wants to change it," while treating symptoms with home remedies: gargling with salt water, a plant called *divedive, chayota* water, or lemon with baking soda. Describing these remedies, Andreina became animated and told me about a naturopathic doctor she loved named Dr. Aristedes who worked out of a storefront in Santa Teresa. She said, "It's great, a lot of people go because this doctor just by looking at you knows what you are suffering from. And he heals you and he personally prepares the medicine." Andreina, a government-trained health promoter for Barrio Adentro, sought care from a naturopath who diagnosed patients without taking their history or conducting an exam. She seemed untroubled by her admiration for two seemingly contradictory models of medicine. Andreina's embrace of medical pluralism did not diminish her enthusiasm for government health programs like Barrio Adentro that operated within the biomedical paradigm.

INTEGRATING BARRIO ADENTRO INTO EXISTING HEALTH PRACTICES

I introduced this chapter with Andreina and Nilda because their medical worldview represented that of many research participants. This worldview included the following beliefs:

- Barrio Adentro offered better biomedical care than private clinics and public hospitals.

- Biomedicine was invaluable but potentially dangerous and should be used with caution.

- Biomedicine was only one of many legitimate healing systems.

Most research participants shared an eagerness to take advantage of new biomedical services, worried about the hazards of biomedicine, and continued to use popular medicine for many of their health needs. The lack of government regulation of people's health behaviors and numerous choices for care produced a sense of pleasure and freedom regarding one's health. In the next section I show how poor and working-class people experienced freedom to engage (or not engage) with biomedical care. Then I show how popular medicine continued to thrive in the wake of Barrio Adentro and explain how government officials promoted health practices beyond biomedicine.

"Aprovechando": Making the Most of Biomedicine

Poor and working-class Venezuelans expressed impatience to make the most of government medicine. This attitude ran deeper than the desire to treat medical problems. Among some people I observed a sense of urgency to maximize the benefits of government medicine because it was unavailable in the past. One way to understand this orientation to medical care is by thinking about the word people used to describe what they were doing: *aprovechando.* The verb *aprovechar* carries multiple meanings. At a basic level it means "to use," but its connotations extend beyond a straightforward translation. *Aprovechar* can also mean "to make the most of / take as a benefit," "to enjoy," and "to take advantage of."

María was a middle-aged Barrio Adentro patient and community health worker in Santa Teresa who struggled with epilepsy. Her husband's health problems caused him to walk with a limp and eat a restricted diet. I frequently encountered her at government health events such as outdoor health fairs and on days when Barrio Adentro optometrists visited Santa Teresa to fit people for free eyeglasses. María said that she was lucky because her sister was a doctor in the nearby city of Maracay, so she used to travel there for medical attention or call her sister to ask for "favors." But needing to rely on her sister caused her shame. Now she did not need to embarrass herself by asking for charity because she could take advantage of free health care from the government.

María said, "We go all over the place for medical care. Chávez has set up a lot of great places, and they're all free. You've got to use it!" She added, "Con Chávez, tienes que aprovechar"—"With Chávez, you have to make the most of it." Initially, I thought she was simply explaining her own position on seeking health care. Later I realized she was also offering me advice. The next time I saw María she tried to convince me to *aprovechar* by urging me to get an eye exam and glasses at a neighborhood health fair. I explained that I recently had an eye exam. María dismissed my protest, saying she could tell I was too embarrassed to ask for help myself. She interrupted the optometrist in the middle of an eye exam to explain that I wanted glasses too. For María, it made no sense to fail to take advantage of a free health service.

Throughout my fieldwork, patients, friends, doctors, nurses, and health volunteers urged me to aprovechar Barrio Adentro's services, from plying me with packets of medications and vitamins they thought I might need to confirming I was up-to-date on vaccinations and urging me to complete a routine gynecological exam. One day after observing doctor-patient interactions with Dr. Cardenas he bid me good-bye with a gift of antibiotics, saying he thought I had an infection because I was coughing and seemed to have low energy.

The language of aprovechando, of taking advantage of Barrio Adentro health care, communicated the historical unavailability of government biomedicine. A patient named Amelia reflected the sentiments of many I met when she said to me, "We've *never* had this kind of health care before." When for decades a doctor's visit was something that only the elite could be assured of getting whenever they wanted, going to the doctor signified more than the services themselves. Accessing biomedical care reflected a kind of empowerment for people who had not had such access before. This was exciting and politically significant.

Serena, a third-year medical student, agreed that Barrio Adentro served as a source of pleasure for patients because it represented a new accessibility to care. Serena was a Caraqueña from a working-class family in Santa Teresa doing a placement in her local Barrio Adentro community clinic for her medical degree. During an interview she began talking about patients who visited clinics for extamedical reasons.

SERENA: Look, you can go to any of these clinics like you see here and you'd see in almost all of these clinics the patients who come here every single day.

AMY: Why?

SERENA: Because "My head hurts," because "Look I found a little round lump here," because "Today I woke up with a foot ache." Any old thing. Because [before] the hunger for health care was so great that now people go to the doctor for the simple satisfaction of knowing they will be taken care of.

Serena cited the historical "hunger for health care" that poor and working-class Venezuelans experienced and the "satisfaction" they felt at having that hunger addressed by government doctors in the present. Patients felt satisfaction that exceeded medicine itself. In Serena's view, patients enjoyed daily confirmation that they could obtain health care whenever they wanted it.

Patients who celebrated the freedom to aprovechar government health care tended to describe these services as widely available, even abundant, but the experience of accessing health care was more uneven. Enthusiasm about accessing new health services overlapped with unrealistic assumptions that the oil-rich government could provide for all as long as people sought out services. One day, during a conversation with two neighborhood residents in a waiting room full of Barrio Adentro patients, the community health worker Magdalena claimed, "Anything you need you can ask for it in Miraflores and you will get it!" Another time, as I spoke with a patient who was telling me about the state health institutions that her family used, she stated categorically, "If someone's not getting [medical care], it's because they don't want it." This attitude was widespread among Caraqueños who viewed Barrio Adentro in a positive light. Research participants told me about people on the Metro begging for money to pay for medical care and passengers telling them to go to Barrio Adentro rather than ask for charity. As I rode the Metro with a community health worker named Clara, we watched a man begging for money to pay for medications. Clara leaned into me and whispered, "If it was really medicine he wanted, he could just go to Barrio Adentro."

Perceptions that state health services could satisfy all medical needs if patients sought them out obscured a complicated reality. In spite of improvements in recent years, in 2008 Venezuelan public medicine remained fractured and incomplete. Long-standing problems with public hospitals and the government's focus on primary and preventive care meant that specialized care suffered. Recall Andreina's story of submitting petitions for government offices to pay private clinics for surgeries and other specialized care. On a daily basis, dozens of people sat patiently under a tent on the grounds of Miraflores, waiting in the sweltering heat to submit or follow up on a petition for presidential assistance. Each month thousands of people appealed to the president via newspaper classifieds and Twitter for help with urgent medical problems, evidencing a large pool of individuals with unmet health needs in spite of a vastly expanded medical system.[11]

And not everyone viewed medicine as something to aprovechar. While some patients visited Barrio Adentro at the first sign of a cold or stomachache, others waited until their problem progressed to an unbearable level of discomfort before seeking care. Medical professionals complained about patients who ignored advice about medications, failed to adopt diet and exercise recommendations, and put off preventive care. Cuban doctors complained that Venezuelans did not do everything they should to optimize their health. Venezuelan patients with asthma or hypertension were not as vigilant as they should be; pregnant woman did not submit to control (prenatal monitoring) with the frequency doctors desired. Cuban doctors' perceptions of patient behavior were shaped by their experiences on the island, where patients had long been encouraged to rely on the country's family doctor program for any possible health concern.[12] While patients expressed enthusiasm about making the most of Barrio Adentro services and national data showed millions more doctors' visits than in previous years, a shift to increased biomedical care seeking was not totalizing.

Biomedical Caution

Widespread caution about certain aspects of biomedicine limited the extent to which people used government services. Reluctance to embrace biomedicine was most apparent in how people used pharmaceuticals.

Access to pharmaceuticals skyrocketed in the first decade of the 2000s as Barrio Adentro increased the supply of and demand for medications. Now with easy access to doctors, people discovered they had been living with chronic diseases for years, undiagnosed. Asthma, diabetes, and hypertension were the most common diseases affecting Barrio Adentro patients, all of which could require lifetime pharmaceutical management. And because of Barrio Adentro, poor and working-class people gained access to medications for these and other problems as never before. The program supplied over one hundred types of prescription medications for free. According to one study, Barrio Adentro had 1,441 tons of medication at its disposal in its first year of operation and doctors distributed 13 million prescription medications.[13] Beyond the free medications provided by the revolutionary government, pharmaceutical sales also increased dramatically in the first decade of the 2000s. From 1998 to 2008, annual pharmaceutical sales increased from 14 to 22 packets per person.[14]

An interview with Viki (a nursing student) and Katerina (Viki's friend and my research assistant) reflects commonsense understandings of how Barrio Adentro changed pharmaceutical use in Venezuela.

KATERINA: Do you think people's use of pharmaceuticals has increased in Venezuela since the founding of Barrio Adentro?

VIKI: Yes, of course. Absolutely.

KATERINA: So people are using medications more than before?

VIKI: *Ufff!* So much more, because now they get them for free, now they have the opportunity to do so. Before they couldn't because they couldn't buy them.

In my structured clinical observations of more than 170 doctor-patient interactions in Santa Teresa's Barrio Adentro clinics,[15] patients left with packets of medication in 40 percent of all visits and 10 percent of patients received a prescription for a medication not available in the clinic. Viki was right to think that medication use had skyrocketed: the proliferation of pharmaceutical use after Barrio Adentro made Venezuela the highest per capita consumer of pharmaceuticals in Latin America in 2008.[16]

During this period, multinational pharmaceutical companies began expanding their reach into poor and working-class communities in Venezuela. In 2007 Pfizer began training barrio residents to become pharmaceutical representatives, which resulted in a 300 percent increase in market share for their drug Lipitor in the sprawling Caracas barrio of Petare in spite of the fact that the drug sold in Venezuela for up to one-fourth of the monthly income for minimum-wage earners.[17]

Amidst this pharmaceutical surge, Caraqueños expressed ambivalence about prescription drugs. People fretted about the risks of counterfeit drugs and even worried about generic drugs manufactured with low-quality ingredients. The risk of purchasing counterfeit pharmaceuticals in Venezuela was serious enough to warrant a public health campaign featuring posters in clinics telling patients how to protect themselves.

Research participants described pharmaceuticals pejoratively as "chemicals" or "chemically based." The chemical (hence, unnatural) properties of pharmaceuticals, in conjunction with the industrial processes involved in their production, rendered pharmaceuticals unknowable and ambiguously powerful, capable of bringing benefits, causing harm, or doing both simultaneously.

Often when people expressed concerns about the ambiguous powers of pharmaceuticals they stated these concerns indirectly in discussions of "natural medicines," which they set in opposition to pharmaceuticals. Natural medicine included herbs and other plants that were unprocessed or minimally processed and were derived from clearly identifiable botanical, or "natural," sources. The assumption was that by their very nature, natural medicines were inherently safe; even if they did not cure a certain problem, they would not do harm.

Negotiations over the appropriateness of "chemical" versus "natural" medicines reflected caution about prescription biomedical treatments that were now available on a widespread basis. Zoraida, a middle-class government administrator, explained her concerns that pharmaceuticals caused more harm than good.

> As a country, we are starting to realize that the big foreign companies have invaded with their chemical medications, that in recent years we've had a greater incidence of cancer [as a result], and have discovered that many medications that treat one symptom can cause harm to a different part of the body. Many people are starting to realize this. And others, we've been raised with the knowledge of plants from our own mothers, you know? I love [botanical medicine]. This doesn't mean I won't take some other kind of medicine sometime. But I love . . . what you can do with . . . plants. And for babies, it's really important to take care of them and give them plants instead of giving them chemicals.

Though many expressed excitement about Barrio Adentro, biomedical pharmaceuticals were by no means the obvious or preferred choice. They stirred up anxieties of bodily harm and financial exploitation. Zoraida claimed pharmaceuticals were the harmful product of invasive foreign capital while viewing natural medicines in terms of romantic images of local flora and familial intimacies. In spite of their status as the top regional consumer of pharmaceuticals, Venezuelans expressed concerns about their potency and carefully negotiated their use. What Caraqueños said about pharmaceuticals revealed that they felt significant freedom with regard to how and to what extent they engaged with biomedicine. They often relied on popular healing practices imagined to be less dangerous and closer to nature than biomedical treatments.

BEYOND BIOMEDICINE

Gaining access to biomedicine through Barrio Adentro did not diminish people's use of popular medical practices such as spiritual healing and natural medicine. Caraqueños usually combined treatments from different healing traditions to cure sickness or to boost well-being, and this did not change as biomedical services expanded during the first decade of the 2000s. People did not change their health practices to become fully biomedical subjects, nor did the Bolivarian government encourage them to. In fact, Chávez and other government officials framed all kinds of health seeking as a means of empowerment and endorsed popular healing practices as valuable alternatives to biomedicine.

Medical traditions in Venezuela loosely mapped onto social hierarchies of class, gender, and ethnicity. Many nonbiomedical traditions such as *espiritismo, santería,* and plant-based medicine carried associations with historically marginalized groups, including indigenous people, poor people, women, and Afro-Venezuelans. However, the esteem that accrued to different medical systems was not determined by their status in the medical hierarchy or by their association with particular social groups.[18]

Spiritual healing traditions included religious practices related to Catholicism, Pentecostalism, and Seventh Day Adventism and syncretic religious traditions such as espiritismo (also known as the cult of María Lionza; autochthonous to Venezuela) and santería (which originated in Cuba).[19] Espiritismo synthesized indigenous, Afro-Venezuelan, folk Catholic, and Kardecist spiritist beliefs in a practice involving different spirit courts to which practitioners appealed via mediums.[20] Venezuelans commonly practiced more than one form of spiritual healing. Although 90 percent of the country was nominally Catholic, researchers estimated that between 30 and 80 percent of Venezuelans subscribed to another form of spiritual healing, such as espiritismo.[21]

Venezuelans complemented spiritual healing and biomedicine with popular empirical medicine. "Empirical medicine" refers to health practices rooted

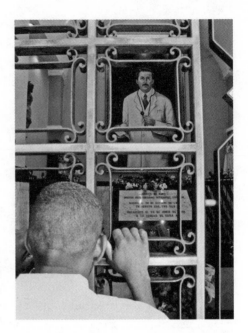

FIGURE 10. Devotee praying in front
of José Gregorio Hernández's remains,
Iglesia de la Candelaria, 2008.
Photo by the author.

in observation and experience of the treatment's effects (as opposed to belief
in a spiritual power). Venezuelans of all social classes relied on home remedies, herbal infusions, and traditional foods to heal illness and promote
health. Many sought out specialists in natural medicine for care. Asian-
derived health practices such as yoga, acupuncture, and meditation were also
popular among people of all social classes.

The boundaries between biomedicine and popular medicine were blurry
and porous in Venezuela (and Latin America more broadly). Biomedical
practitioners incorporated knowledge from popular empirical medicine (e.g.,
home remedies, homeopathy, plant-based medicine) into their work with
patients. Popular healers incorporated knowledge and symbolism from biomedicine into their practices. The beloved doctor turned popular saint José
Gregorio Hernández underlines the permeable boundaries between biomedicine and popular healing. Devotees frequented his shrine in the
Catholic church in Caracas that held his remains (fig. 10). The cult of María
Lionza relied on José Gregorio's spirit to preside over its medical "court,"
consisting of famous long-dead Venezuelan doctors. José Gregorio was ubiquitous in hospitals as well, appearing in shrines, portraits hanging on the
walls, and at patients' bedsides. Meanwhile, "mystical hospitals" and spiritist
clinics in barrios provided spiritual cures with the simulacra of high-tech

biomedical centers.[22] The anthropologist Francisco Ferrándiz conducted fieldwork in the mid-1990s in a mystical hospital that treated over six hundred patients a week via surgeries conducted by the spirits of famous doctors, in a setting and with procedures that resembled those of an actual hospital, including nurses wearing uniforms, patient charts and files, and post-"operation" bandages. Patients kept their bandages until they returned to the hospital to remove the symbolic stitches a week later.[23]

Research participants did not view this lively medical pluralism as exceptional or problematic; rather, it was the expected norm. We can see how this played out at the individual level by recalling Nilda, her mother, and Andreina and their health practices. Medical pluralism also characterized Luisa's approach to health. Luisa was a member of Santa Teresa's Grandparents Club, but she did not live in Santa Teresa. She used a cane to navigate rickety buses, hills, narrow sidewalks, and potholes to travel from the barrio of El Valle to the high school where the club met for dance therapy. Luisa preferred this club because she liked its energy and the fact that it met five days a week. The day I met Luisa I observed her in discussion with another club member, debating a salve Luisa purchased in a popular medicine store. Luisa planned to use it on her knee. Her friend dismissed the salve, saying it wouldn't work as well as cut onions placed on the knee overnight. Using onions in this way was a *remedio casero,* or home remedy, that I had heard people discuss before.

Learning I was a foreigner, Luisa drew my attention to the brooch she was wearing. It displayed a likeness of José Gregorio Hernández. "He was a doctor in Venezuela, and now he's a saint. He performs miracles," Louisa explained matter-of-factly. She once suffered from what doctors said was an incurable illness of the legs and spinal column. Every night she prayed to José Gregorio, placed his image under a glass of water, and drank the water in the morning. She healed herself this way and afterward became a *devota,* or devotee, of the doctor-saint.

When I told her I was in Venezuela to study health care she became animated. "I use Barrio Adentro a lot. They are great doctors! It's a wonderful program," Luisa volunteered. She used to use the Military Hospital because her husband had been in the military, but if she hadn't had access there, she said she would not have had anywhere to go before. "How dare the [private] doctors here charge 200 bolivares [approximately US$90]? How can they do that?," she demanded, suggesting that she could not afford such a visit and that to charge so much was an outrage. Luisa visited a Barrio Adentro clinic that very day to get a doctor's note attesting to her hearing loss so she could take it to the mayor's office for free hearing aids.

In this brief conversation, Luisa mentioned participating in five separate health practices in the past twenty-four hours: dance therapy with the Grandparents Club, using a popular medicinal salve, praying to a popular saint, seeking care from Barrio Adentro, and petitioning the mayor's office for a medical device. She also discussed the pros and cons of other health practices: home remedies, seeking care from a state hospital, and going to a private practice physician. Luisa's diverse health practices drew from biomedical, spiritual, and popular empirical systems. Like other Caraqueños, Luisa engaged in these health practices thoughtfully and agentively.

The forms of medical pluralism I observed in the first decade of the 2000s paralleled the Venezuelan practices that the anthropologist Angelina Pollak-Eltz described twenty years earlier, in the early 1980s.

> Maybe 60% of all diseases and minor ailments are treated at home with well-known remedies. . . . [W]hen the illness gets worse, friends and relatives may be consulted . . . [and] people may resort to stronger remedies such as antibiotics, which they prescribe themselves. Others stick to old-fashioned herbal remedies, prescribed by older relatives. . . . When the illness is treated at home, candles may be burned for José Gregorio Hernández or other saints and a vow may be made, to be paid for as soon as the person recovers. If the illness gets worse and the patient decides to get help from a specialist, he has many options: 1) . . . a doctor in the local health center . . . [;] 2) a doctor in a [Social Security clinic], provided he is covered . . . [;] 3) . . . a doctor in a church-sponsored clinic, the Red Cross or another institution . . . [;] 4) . . . a private doctor . . . [whose] fees are high . . . [;] 5) . . . [or] the patient may travel to the United States or Europe for further consultations. This option is of course limited only to those who can afford such trips. 6) . . . a local herbalist . . . [;] 7) . . . a spiritual healer[;]' 8) . . . services in the centers of the Cult of Maria Lionza . . . [;] 9) . . . a faith healer in the Pentecostal church.[24]

With a few changes this list could describe Venezuelan health practices in the 2000s. Of course, the introduction of Barrio Adentro in poor and working-class neighborhoods made it the first choice of biomedical care for many people. And although I did not meet anyone who had traveled to Europe or North America for treatments, I did know people who traveled to Cuba for free eye surgeries. While Barrio Adentro allowed people to avoid less attractive options like visiting a hospital or private clinic, self-medicating with pharmaceuticals, and adopting a wait-and-see approach, nobody reported using popular medicine any less because Barrio Adentro was available.

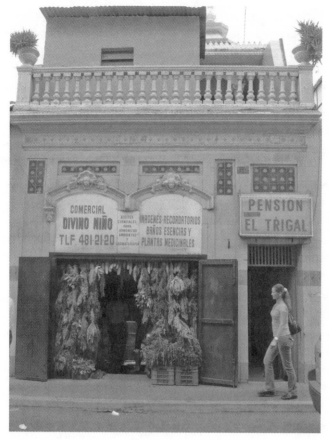

FIGURE 11. Shop specializing in popular medicine, 2008. Photo by the author.

If anything, biomedical alternatives proliferated when the government instituted Barrio Adentro. Observations I made suggest that people became more engaged with popular medical practices during the early 2000s. In late 2008 I conducted interviews with workers in the shops specializing in popular medicine on Avenida Baralt. This street demarcated the western perimeter of Santa Teresa and was known by city residents as an important place to get personalized treatments and popular healing products (fig. 11).[25] Of the sixteen shops I surveyed that specialized in popular medicine, half had been in business for twenty years or more while the other half opened after Chávez became president. Shopkeepers agreed that their businesses were unaffected by the doubling of local competition or by the expansion of Barrio Adentro.

They said that over the past five years customer interest in popular medicine had increased and that in spite of increased competition their businesses were doing as well as before or better. Some told me that Cuban *santería* and herbal medicine in particular were booming.

Other evidence confirmed shopkeepers' claims that Caraqueños were more engaged in these practices since the advent of Barrio Adentro. Claims of rising sales of santería supplies matched claims from residents of Santa Teresa, some of whom were themselves believers, about the increasing popularity of the Afro-Cuban religion. During my fieldwork Venezuelans' interest in santería attracted media attention and academic commentary, with one journalist reporting that in the past five years the number of stores dedicated to santería in the city doubled to over 150 shops.[26]

Regarding claims about a rise in plant-based medicine, I interviewed a group of medicinal plant vendors from El Junquito, a rural area near Caracas, who said their business has boomed since 2001 when they began supplying herbs for empirical and spiritual healing to the shops along Avenida Baralt. As we talked we stood next to their pickup truck, the bed piled high with bundles of different plants, all cut to arm's length. In seven years' time their business multiplied, requiring them to upgrade from a four-door car to a pickup truck and a van for biweekly deliveries to the city. During that period the team was the exclusive vendor of plants from this region, suggesting that local demand rather than a reduction in competition drove rising sales.

Observations from the Catholic Church of la Candelaria in central Caracas suggested a possible increase in the numbers of devotees to José Gregorio Hernández. People flocked to the site of his remains to pray for healing and good health. Vendors outside the church who sold religious objects related to José Gregorio (including plaster figurines, healing balms, and *estampitas,* cards featuring his image and a prayer) all reported observing more devotees visiting the church in recent years. Two of the six vendors began working there in the past three years, suggesting a rise in consumption of spiritual healing products sufficient to support new competition.

GOVERNMENT SUPPORT FOR MEDICAL PLURALISM

Wondering why people used biomedical alternatives (perhaps at higher rates than before) during a historic expansion of government biomedicine invokes the question of why people use popular medicine at all. One commonly held belief is that people rely on popular medicine only when presumably more modern and effective biomedical care is unavailable.[27] The assumption that when given a choice people will naturally prefer biomedicine does not stand up to cross-cultural scrutiny. In Latin America the emergence and consolidation of professional biomedicine in the nineteenth and twentieth centuries did not diminish forms of popular healing and may have had the opposite effect; that is, it may have contributed to a flourishing of alternative healing practices.[28]

Another theory is that people turn to popular medicine—especially spiritual healing—during economic and political unrest to relieve anxiety and anxiety-induced bodily complaints. Other anthropologists suggest this explanation to account for the numbers of devotees of José Gregorio Hernández and the cult of María Lionza before and during the Chávez presidency.[29] But viewing popular medical practices as cultural responses to the distress of political and economic upheaval makes little sense in this case. Research participants viewed the period of Chávez's presidency as an era of optimism and empowerment, not as a time of social trauma.[30] Their perspective was the majority view in Venezuela at that time. Based on surveys from the period 2006–9, 80 percent of Venezuelans reported satisfaction with their standard of living and 90 percent reported satisfaction with their personal health.[31] Income inequality was falling while the country's ranking in the United Nations Human Development Index was rising.[32] I met many Venezuelans who expressed anxiety about Chávez-era changes in society and politics, but they rarely belonged to Caracas's poor or working classes.

We must address another assumption, that medicine fundamentally functions to cure illness. We often assume that people use medicine—whether popular medicine or biomedicine—to solve problems. But popular medical practices in Latin America commonly promote health and wellness in the absence of a specific pathology. People seek out traditional local foods known to bring joy, comfort, and health benefits. People like Nilda use acupuncture or yoga to maintain a state of "balance" and a sense of well-being in the world. Devotees pray to José Gregorio in times of health and in times of illness. The potential for medicine to serve not just a curative function but also as a source of meaning and pleasure is not unique to the Venezuelan context. Farquhar's ethnographic research on Chinese traditional medicine reveals that people derived great pleasure from it. She advises us to stop assuming that people only use medicine to resolve problems.

Too often in anthropology the mere existence of a cultural institution, such as a group of practices known as an 'alternative medicine,' is enough to persuade us that there must be some basic and universal human need that this set of practices functions to fulfill. . . . [Instead] I want to consider some of the pleasures that may be cultivated by those who . . . seek traditional medical care. Although it may seem odd to think of medical services as objects of desire, as fulfilling wants rather than needs, perhaps in the case of Chinese medicine and its positive view of health this is not so far-fetched.[33]

Popular medicine flourished after the advent of Barrio Adentro for many reasons. Recognizing that biomedicine and popular medicine almost always coexist and that medicine does more than treat distress suggests that we should not be surprised by a lively commitment to medical pluralism in Caracas. In addition, unique historical conditions encouraged people to engage in pluralistic health seeking. For one thing, high global oil prices boosted the country's economy during this period, enabling people to spend more on popular medical practices than in other eras.

Another factor that played a role in people's health behaviors was the revolutionary government's endorsement of health seeking in all its forms—including popular medicine—as a means to happiness and empowerment. Under Chávez, the government expanded health services and encouraged poor and working-class Venezuelans to take care of their health as a way to demarginalize themselves. State institutions fostered expectations for good health and legitimated health beliefs and behaviors that were already circulating. The 1999 Constitution, which people enthusiastically endorsed and frequently quoted verbatim during my fieldwork, framed access to health care as a basic human right guaranteed by the state and supported by the participatory governance of ordinary people. Articles 83–85 explain guarantees of health:

> Health is a fundamental social right and the responsibility of the State. . . . All persons have the right to protection of health, as well as the duty to participate actively in the furtherance and protection of the same. . . .
>
> In order to guarantee the right to health, the State creates, exercises guidance over and administers a national public health system that . . . is decentralized and participatory in nature . . . governed by principles of gratuity, universality, completeness, fairness, social integration and solidarity. . . .
>
> The organized community has the right and duty to participate in making decisions concerning policy planning, implementation, and control of public health institutions.[34]

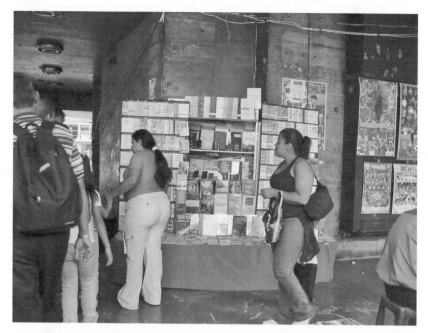

FIGURE 12. Street vendor selling printed laws, 2006. Photo by the author.

Many Venezuelans could recite parts of the 1999 Constitution from memory, and street vendors made a living by selling printed laws (fig. 12). As one woman explained, "Before the state treated people very badly. That is starting to change. The language of the people is changing, too. Now they are reading the constitution."

Barrio Adentro and other social projects were efforts to make good on constitutional promises to uphold a right to health care. The government's expansion of health services encouraged people to expect that if they sought out health care they would receive it. Research participants assured me this represented a new reality for them.

Government institutions encouraged health seeking by expanding health education. Health education included public service announcements, free books and pamphlets on health topics, exercise programs for schoolchildren and older adults, health promoter training, and professional medical training targeted at members of historically marginalized communities.

While encouraging poor and working-class Venezuelans to take heed of their right to health, the Chávez government remained agnostic about the superiority of different healing systems. Government institutions encouraged people to practice biomedical alternatives, even offering some of these in their own clinics. Barrio Adentro Rehabilitation Centers (SRIs) provided physical and speech therapy as well as acupuncture, magnetic healing, and hydrotherapy. Dr. Cardenas, the Venezuelan physician who worked in one of Santa Teresa's Barrio Adentro clinics, prescribed homeopathic formulas in addition to pharmaceuticals. Courses offered by the National Institute of Geriatrics included topics such as health promotion through natural and traditional local foods. The facilitator of one course was a naturopath named Paulina who commented that in twenty years of practicing natural medicine, this government was the most supportive of biomedical alternatives.

The Bolivarian government set legal precedents to incorporate popular medicine into officially sanctioned medical practice in Venezuela. The 1999 Constitution recognized the value of popular medicine in Venezuela, framed in terms of indigenous rights. Article 122 states, "Native peoples have the right to a full health system that takes into consideration their practices and cultures. The State shall recognize their traditional medicine and complementary forms of therapy, subject to the principles of bioethics."[35] In 2001, the government created the National Commission of Complementary Therapies (CONATEC), which lawmakers described as follows:

> A permanent group that will advise the Ministry of Health and Social Development in the analysis, revision, development of standards, implementation, and evaluation of complementary therapies. . . . The Health and Social Development Ministry will encourage scientific research in the field and create a database that will allow expansion, evaluation, and follow-up regarding the program.[36]

When activists for traditional and complementary medicine met with legislators working on health laws in 2008, one lawmaker assured them of continued government support for popular medicine, saying, "The deputies on this subcommittee unanimously offer our resounding support to all of traditional medicine and complementary therapies. . . . After all, who has not benefited from natural medicines?"[37]

The government's hospitable stance toward popular medical traditions was not without precedent in Latin America. Although biomedical hegemony and attempts to marginalize popular medical traditions have been the historical norm, recently governments have promoted the concept of intercultural health.

Intercultural health policies integrate popular medical healers and practices with biomedical service networks to improve health outcomes, specifically, among rural and indigenous populations.[38] Most governments implement the notion of intercultural health in a piecemeal fashion to improve health indicators rather than as a means of recognition and empowerment. But Bolivia and Ecuador, like Venezuela, went a step further and formally recognized popular medical traditions by revising their constitutions and establishing government bodies to address indigenous health/traditional medicine. It is not coincidence that Bolivia, Ecuador, and Venezuela each became more supportive of popular medicine under the leadership of socialist presidents whose politics focused on empowering poor and indigenous people.

By endorsing rather than delegitimizing biomedical alternatives, the Chávez government empowered social groups historically associated with these medical practices. Official support for popular medicine reflected pragmatism about the cultural importance of these traditions and showed respect for the people who valued them. Officials and public service announcements exhorted Venezuelans to use Barrio Adentro and other health programs, but they did not frame biomedicine as the triumph of modernism over traditionalism, as other Latin American governments have done. Rather, government officials—including Chávez—went on record praising the unique healing powers of popular medicine.

PLEASURE AND POWER BEYOND BIOMEDICINE

To summarize, the Chávez government transformed people's experience of medical pluralism in three ways that produced pleasure and empowerment.

First, the government invested heavily in biomedical services like Barrio Adentro, leading to a proliferation in the number of sites offering health care. Opening thousands of biomedical sites altered the landscape of medical pluralism in Venezuela and improved people's ability to choose biomedicine. Previously, poor and working-class Venezuelans might have desired biomedical services but been unable to use them due to barriers of cost and distance. A sense of empowerment resulted from experiencing greater agency to access biomedicine.

Second, the idiosyncrasies and partiality of Venezuela's reforms produced few restrictions on how people engaged with state health services. People took pleasure knowing they could visit any of Barrio Adentro's preventive care clinics, directly access a diagnostic center or hospital, and appeal to a special medical fund. Regardless of whether this reflected an intentional policy, research participants commented on the sense of freedom that a laissez-faire organization of government medicine provided. It allowed them to choose a clinic for reasons as varied as location, doctor's personality, clinic reputation, or access to high-tech equipment. With the exception of scarce specialist services, people usually accessed government biomedicine as frequently as they wanted, as no system was in place to prevent patients from revisiting a neighborhood clinic over and over or from obtaining diagnostic tests or treatments from multiple sites. The organization (or lack of organization) of government health care led some people to feel they had an excess of choices for biomedical services.

The government also made no effort to mandate population health, leaving people free to completely disengage from encounters with state biomedicine if they wished. Although Barrio Adentro used Cuban administrators and doctors to implement a Cuban model of health care, the Venezuelan government did not consolidate control over people's health practices as Cuba did. By design, Cuba's Family Doctor program collected detailed data on a block-by-block basis to develop individualized plans that promoted healthy behaviors. Christina Perez's ethnographic research shows how doctors and nurses cared for the people in their neighborhood catchment area, including gathering information and classifying every resident's risk factors through a policy known as *dispensarización*.[39] Referring specifically to this practice, the Cuban health care scholar Julie Feinsilver claimed that "the fundamental task of the family doctor [was] to aggressively investigate and monitor the entire population."[40] This comprehensive management of population health was absent from Barrio Adentro medical care. Barrio Adentro workers did not track the neighborhood's health or even keep charts on patients.[41]

Third, government officials formally recognized and promoted respect for popular medical traditions. They never presented Barrio Adentro as a replacement for existing health practices, nor did they try to delegitimize popular medicine. In fact, government officials encouraged people to continue practicing medical pluralism. The government's positive attitude to medical pluralism communicated that poor and working-class Venezuelans enjoyed agency and control over their own health practices. Research participants felt free to critique and reject biomedical treatments based on cultural logics of health. This made government medicine easier to use than it might have been otherwise and led people to view the Chávez government and its health programs as allied with their desires, beliefs, and ways of life.

Comparing Venezuelan and Cuban approaches to medical pluralism underlines the political ramifications of government responses to popular healing traditions. For decades, socialist Cuba consolidated biomedical authority by delegitimizing popular medicine.[42] The anthropologist Sean Brotherton explains:

> The [Cuban] state's narrowly defined vision of science and development in the health sector meant a disavowal of alternative perspectives and approaches to biomedical health care. For example, the role of midwives, *curanderos* (traditional healers), syncretic-based religions such as Santería, and natural and traditional medicine, among other alternatives to biomedicine, were actively marginalized and effectively criminalized as "occult sciences" by the socialist government.[43]

By practicing dispensarización in neighborhood clinics and working to curtail popular medical practices, the Cuban state sought to achieve population health and reshape people's ideas and practices in favor of biomedical approaches. While aiming to empower Cubans by eradicating diseases and promoting scientific understandings of the body, government policies sent a message that alternative perspectives offered little of value (and could even produce harm). According to Brotherton, the Cuban state inculcated in people a biomedicalized view of bodies and health that became so dominant that in the 1990s, when economic crises forced government clinics to replace biomedical treatments with plant-based and Asian medicine, patients rejected them as inferior substitutes.[44]

Government support for popular medical traditions empowered Venezuelans by ceding control of health practices to the people and by valuing and dignifying medical traditions historically associated with marginalized social groups. When a government or other authoritative institution devalues or delegitimizes a popular medical tradition, it devalues and delegitimizes the people associated with this tradition (regardless of whether individuals in this social group subscribe to it). Official efforts to undermine particular medical systems communicate that users and practitioners are threats to progress and unready for nation-state belonging. If governments improve people's access to hegemonic forms of medicine—usually biomedicine—without interfering with how they engage in other medical traditions, they send a very different message. By valuing and legitimizing popular medicine, they also value and legitimize historically marginalized social groups. By supporting the country's lively medical pluralism, government policies produced meaningful experiences of agency and recognition beyond biomedical care.

FIVE

Pleasures of Participation

IN THIS CHAPTER AND THE FOLLOWING CHAPTER, I shift focus from individuals seeking medical care in revolutionary Venezuela to analyze what happened when groups of people cooperated on health promotion projects in public settings. Under Chávez, government health promotion projects encouraged ordinary citizens to participate in activities designed to improve their health or the health of other people who lived in their neighborhood. This chapter describes people's experiences of community health work and elderly exercise clubs, two of the most popular forms of health promotion. Having observed the immense popularity of these activities, I wanted to examine why people participated in them with such enthusiasm. My research revealed that participants derived pleasure not only from working on bodily health but also from transforming the meanings of community public spaces. Whether wearing the bright red attire of pro-government activism or performing bailoterapia in an otherwise derelict plaza, people enjoyed a sense of empowerment and visibility while collaborating to revitalize themselves and their neighborhoods.

Community health promotion enabled a culturally valued form of participation among people who previously felt they had no stake in public life. Research participants viewed the government's call to participate in these programs as an opportunity for them to thrive rather than as a means for the Bolivarian government to cynically achieve its own goals via the efforts of individual citizens. Poor and working-class people who joined these programs emphasized that they had felt excluded from formal politics until these programs came along, offering them substantive roles in society and politics. Participants said that such opportunities were unavailable elsewhere and impossible to develop on their own without government support.

Activists in Training

People took pleasure in government health care not only as patients but also as activists. To keep its health programs running, Barrio Adentro relied on ordinary people to work as unpaid community health workers. In many parts of the world community health workers are people who belong to the communities where they provide health care and education. They usually do not have prior medical training. Though this work often took the form of monotonous clinic assistance, Venezuelan community health workers were enthusiastic in their conviction that they were helping redress social inequalities. By training and working as a Barrio Adentro community health worker myself, I documented how promoting health for others served as a source of pleasure. At public events—neighborhood health fairs, for example—volunteers displayed their status as health promoters proudly, making sure they wore Barrio Adentro T-shirts and baseball caps. In private settings I observed volunteers enjoying the shared experience of learning about health promotion.

For twelve weeks a group of Santa Teresa residents (all women) and I met in a Barrio Adentro clinic to complete a voluntary training course in community health.[1] Each Monday we sat in red plastic chairs around Mercedes, the Cuban doctor who cared for the area's patients and mentored its medical students and community health workers. Over her shoulder, a poster encouraged visitors to learn the signs of dengue fever, concluding with the emotional appeal, "In Bolivarian socialism your health is important!" Mercedes tossed out questions to assess our knowledge of the week's topic. "How do you diagnose hypertension?," she would ask, or "What kinds of behaviors suggest a drinking problem?" She encouraged us to share our online research on topics such as obesity, sexually transmitted diseases, and the dangers of smoking, correcting us and answering questions. Classes felt more like friends meeting for book club discussions than government training sessions. While covering the mandatory topics in our module and discussing how to share this knowledge with neighbors, family, and friends, we exchanged personal stories about common health problems. The group shared intimate moments that were alternately playful, like when Mercedes confessed that McDonald's was her guilty pleasure, and sobering, like when Paulita admitted she went fifteen years without a gynecological exam because she did not have access to health care.

Participation in these training sessions was not required in order to become a community health worker, nor were participants rewarded beyond the knowledge and gratification gained in the course. Most in my group had completed at least one Barrio Adentro training program and wanted to do more. When attending classes, the women were fully present in the moment. They diligently produced pages of handwritten notes based on internet research and took turns reading to one another. But they all had other obligations that made weekly attendance difficult. They worked to support their families while also acting as primary caregivers for children and elderly parents. Mercedes chided trainees for their irregular attendance, but the women rarely expressed remorse. Beyond Mercedes's scolding, participants suffered no repercussions for unreliable attendance or even for dropping out.

The week the course ended, I ran into Andreina on the street. Because of a misunderstanding about meeting times, she missed our final class. She said she was disappointed; she had prepared a reference book she wanted to show us. From her handbag she produced a thick scrapbook-style album that she paid to have bound at an office supply store. Andreina spent three days making it. The album covered each course theme, with newspaper clippings and educational pamphlets collected from government offices glued on white paper. The book was impressive. It was far more effort than Mercedes expected of us. The album revealed the extent of Andreina's intellectual curiosity about health promotion and the satisfaction she derived from the training.

Training courses were only one aspect of community health work. Volunteers' main responsibility entailed working in Barrio Adentro primary care clinics one morning a week. According to the Barrio Adentro administration, every primary care clinic needed a Health Committee (Comité de Salud) composed of ten to fifteen local volunteers. These community health workers helped medical staff by maintaining a waiting list of patients; keeping patients company; providing information about health and social services; conducting inventories of medication, bandages, and vaccines; and cleaning the clinic. Some community health workers learned to weigh patients, take blood pressure, and administer injections. Because neighborhood clinics had no employees besides doctors and nurses (sometimes dentists), community health workers played crucial roles in their everyday functioning.

Motivated by the government's uplifting promises and investment in social programs, huge numbers of people joined state-sponsored activist movements in the early 2000s (fig. 13).[2] Among these movements, which included community councils and urban land committees, health activism generated enormous participation. In the first five years after the institution of Barrio Adentro, over 140,000 volunteers founded more than 8,500 health

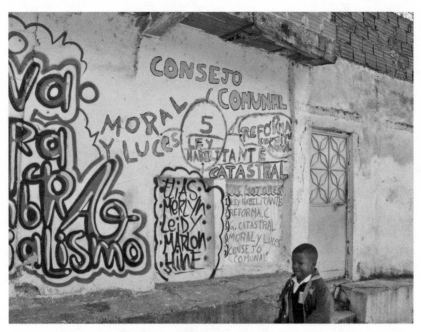

FIGURE 13. Mural celebrating popular participation and legal reforms in the Chávez era, 2008. Photo by the author.

committees nationwide.[3] To put these numbers in perspective, in a 2006 survey of 500 people from eleven Caracas barrios, 25 percent said they had worked in Barrio Adentro as community health workers.[4]

Santa Teresa's community health workers helped establish their first neighborhood clinic(s) in the early years of the Barrio Adentro program, underlining their importance for the program's existence. Municipal administrators assigned Cuban doctors to live and work in a neighborhood, leaving residents to organize housing, food, and clinical space for them. The ad hoc groups of volunteers who responded to the government's call to host these doctors formed the first Health Committees in the neighborhood. Doctors usually lived with a community health worker's family for their first few years, and clinics were often located in a resident's house or in a repurposed community space. Knowing they played such an important role in getting the new health program off the ground provided volunteers with a sense of purpose and gratification.

The community health workers I knew had not worked in medical settings before joining Barrio Adentro. In Santa Teresa, the typical volunteer was an unemployed or underemployed middle-aged woman (fourteen of the fifteen members I knew were between forty-one and fifty-eight years old). All had children, and most had an educational background of a high school diploma or less. Community health workers' economic situation reflected the class diversity of this neighborhood. A few lived in small but comfortable apartments and could afford to travel for a vacation from time to time, while others were unemployed and struggling to pay the bills. None considered themselves the poorest of the poor in this community.

Rather than experience the work as burdensome or as a sacrifice for the greater good, people enjoyed being health promoters. They entered into it voluntarily for a variety of reasons. Some emphasized the tangible benefits for people they helped as a motivating factor. Some wanted to learn more about medicine. A few said they wanted to reciprocate for the benefits they received from government doctors. They all stated that becoming a health promoter was an opportunity to participate in society that they never had before. This last point seemed especially important—that the government would design programs explicitly to encourage their involvement in community work.

The pleasure that community health workers took in activities like the training course was discernible—if you knew what to look for. Beyond intermittent smiles and laughter, the women did not do anything in these sessions that overtly manifested enjoyment. For the most part, they seemed serious and focused on learning. As a participant observer I did not immediately interpret these activities as productive of pleasure for the women. I had to analyze the experience in the larger context of participants' lives to see that they were electing to do this because it held valuable meanings for their sense of self. The work was fulfilling and satisfying even if the pleasure that accrued was not overtly expressed. The cerebral gratification of embodying the role of community health worker contrasted sharply with the playful "work" of dance therapy in Grandparents Clubs, revealing how participating in government health promotion programs could produce different forms of enjoyment.

Dancing for Health and Fun

In contrast to community health workers, members of Grandparents Clubs displayed overt, unmistakable pleasure in the bodily exertion and playful socializing of their exercise classes. I conducted participant observation for months at a time with one of the two clubs in Santa Teresa, in which the dominant tone of their daily sessions was manifest enjoyment. This enjoyment was not merely bodily and social but also political.

On most days when the club met, an eclectic mix of techno, salsa, *joropo*,[5] and reggaeton reverberated in the covered, open-air courtyard of a high school in Santa Teresa, providing the beat for a group of aging residents, mostly women, who danced with enthusiasm. During the session club members trickled into the workout space that was set back from the street behind a barred entrance, where an informal worker stood guard to provide security. Some people wore sneakers and stretchy athletic clothing and intensified their workout with weights they had made by filling water bottles with sand. Others wore orthopedic shoes and housedresses and supported themselves with a cane or by holding onto a concrete column. Illuminated by the last light of dusk and scattered fluorescent bulbs in the concrete ceiling, the dancers frequently turned to others who were sitting and chatting, exhorting us to get up and dance. Participants sashayed across the courtyard and grabbed one of us by the hand in a joking pretense of dragging us into the rows of dancers. One festive evening, Rosa, a stout woman in her late sixties, came over to the bench where I was sitting and sweeping her arms around her in a show of exhilaration, cried, "I could do this all night! Let's party and dance until 5:00 A.M.!" People laughed in agreement.

In this club, members met weekday afternoons inside the school, considered a safe space in a neighborhood that in spite of its working- and middle-class identity was viewed as a *zona roja,* or red zone, a dangerous area prone to muggings and drug-related violence. Members arrived and departed with little regard for the class's official start and end times and took frequent breaks to gossip on benches. Depending on who was leading that day, exercises consisted of spins, squats, salsa steps, dancing in pairs, or moving in large circles or conga lines. Nobody tried to standardize the music, types of dances, or choreography. Some dancers ignored the leader's cues and literally danced to their own beat, making up steps and turns. Participants smiled and laughed throughout the two hours of moving in time to the loud beat.

In Latin America, records of Grandparents Clubs date to the 1970s and show that they were funded by local governments, charitable donations, and members' contributions.[6] Many have a dedicated physical space in which members meet and conduct activities. As in the Venezuelan clubs I observed, club members in other countries are usually older women. The Venezuelan clubs are based on ones that Cuba instituted in the 1990s as part of a comprehensive "elderly care program."[7] Clubs in other countries are generally not as focused on exercise and health promotion as in Cuba and Venezuela, where the Grandparents Clubs are promoted and organized as an extension of local clinics.

The club I describe in this chapter was one of over five thousand exercise clubs founded since 2003. Loosely affiliated with Barrio Adentro clinics, Grandparents Clubs had between thirty and sixty members ranging in age from fifty to ninety. Once a club was established, its members could seek recognition from the state to receive funding and resources, primarily a sports trainer or physiotherapist to lead classes. Membership in the clubs was free or based on a voluntary contribution (usually the equivalent of a few U.S. dollars every month). Grandparents Clubs lacked bureaucratic structures to circumscribe participation. Any person could walk up to an exercise class and begin participating without completing an application or any other formal procedure. Most aging Caraqueños had an active Grandparents Club or two within walking distance of their homes.

Everyone, including the sports trainers assigned to lead members through their strenuous bailoterapia workouts, knew that Grandparents Clubs were intended to do more than boost biophysical health. The clubs were also designed to promote socializing among members and improve psychological well-being. Because of their voluntary nature and the spirit with which club members took up the government's call to participate, the work of becoming healthy felt exhilarating and rewarding.

At first glance, the experiences of community health workers and Grandparents Club members seem unrelated. Community health workers were devoted to other people's health, whereas Grandparents Club members worked on their own health. Community health workers rarely expressed overt pleasure as they worked, whereas Grandparents Club members did so nearly constantly. Yet these seemingly incommensurable experiences of participating in government projects held similar meanings and produced similar outcomes for participants. The activities offered benefits beyond improved biophysical health, namely, opportunities to transform themselves into different kinds of people. Both programs also enabled participants to have positive effects on their community.

PARTICIPATION AS A MEANS OF PERSONAL TRANSFORMATION

Community Health Workers

Community health workers shared a narrative that the revolutionary government motivated them to participate (*participar*) in health activism, which changed how they viewed themselves. They explained that the state's material investment in social services and opportunities for popular participation motivated them to support government health projects that came to their neighborhoods. Lilian, an elected neighborhood official and community health worker, made this point when she told me:

> This is an opportunity that they gave to us so we could organize ourselves, you see? Because before, this didn't exist. They didn't take into account whether someone wanted to be involved. Before what happened was the mayor's office would bring their own personnel to vaccinate and so on, but they didn't take the community into account, there weren't many [community] organizations.

In other words, there was a reciprocal quality to community health work. Only after witnessing material investments in health care did people like Lilian decide to give themselves to community health activism. What drew people to this work were actual government programs providing services, material benefits, and substantive opportunities to effect social change. As Carolina explained, "[I became a volunteer] when the president started to change everything, to make sure that things get to the people who were most in need, like doctors ... people having access to the things that they had never had the opportunity for before."

Magdalena believed that community health work effected a deep personal transformation. As I mentioned in chapter 3, Magdalena decided to volunteer with the Health Committee after her first visit to the Barrio Adentro clinic where a doctor spent time engaging her in a conversation about her health. She said, "[That experience] completely changed me, my way of thinking. I received a benefit, so I participate in the community." She explained undergoing an "awakening" as a community health worker that turned her into "a community person."

MAGDALENA: I became a community person here, in Barrio Adentro.

AMY: You feel like you have changed as a person?

MAGDALENA: Yes, because before, I was very centered on my house. I would leave to shop, to go to church, to visit girlfriends, and then go back to my house again. But with Barrio Adentro you have to attend to the patients and hear about their pains....

It's like an awakening, do you hear me? The truth is there are people in hardship. And the work of [social] promotion is that sometimes I have to lend my legs, my strength, to do what this person cannot do.

If this person cannot move, I have to move for him. It's like, "Love thy neighbor" [Amor al prójimo]. How do you show that you love your neighbor? Put yourself in his place or do the things that he cannot do.

Magdalena described her transformation from being egotistical and individualistic, someone who locks herself up in her house,[8] into a community person, a social promoter. In the excerpt above, she makes two points about this change. She explains her volunteer work as a practice of loving thy neighbor, a biblical reference that many health volunteers (Catholic as well as evangelical) in Santa Teresa used to describe their work in Barrio Adentro. This concept carried significance for Magdalena, a devout evangelical Christian. Government officials during this period also emphasized the importance of love for others as a motivation to fight for social justice. Another interesting part of Magdalena's narrative is the way she explained the mechanism of personal transformation. She claimed to become a person who helps strangers only when she began to provide care to them. Magdalena did not become a health worker because she felt a generosity of spirit or community-mindedness. Rather, through sustained engagement in community health work she found herself becoming the kind of person who embodied the locally salient identity, "community person."

Magdalena punctuated her story of personal transformation with references to her body that physically moved for those whose bodies cannot move and to parts of her body that she metaphorically gave to others ("a shoulder to lean on"; "I lend my legs"). References to bodily movement were relevant for health volunteers who described shifting from a politically passive life of relative self-absorption to an active life of caring for others and engaging in community activism. This personal metamorphosis did not occur instantaneously; rather, it required the adoption of new practices and habits that in their embodiment enabled the individual to become a different type of person.[9]

Magdalena told me that volunteering at the Barrio Adentro clinic was like an awakening: she realized that many people in Santa Teresa needed health care, proper nutrition, and other social services. Community health workers agreed that they only became fully aware of the poverty of fellow residents after they began volunteering in the clinic. This realization motivated them to carry on with their activism, and it motivated some to embark on new careers in social work. Gabriella decided to study community development in the state's new tuition-free Bolivarian University of Venezuela (UBV) after working for Barrio Adentro as a volunteer.

GABRIELLA: What brought me to my current career choice? Barrio Adentro.

AMY: Really?

GABRIELLA: Yes, because I didn't know the hardship in my neighborhood beyond what I saw inside my own apartment building.

AMY: Why do you think you didn't see it before?

GABRIELLA: I didn't have the interest . . . or I had the interest but I was guarded. You know how these things don't become real until you start to focus on them? I would walk down this block, that block, I'd see something grim, but I wouldn't get involved. When I started working with the doctors was when I became aware of all the poverty in this neighborhood. . . . I began working with Barrio Adentro, because they were lacking a nurse. . . . I saw so many in need.

Like Magdalena, Gabriella experienced a personal transformation from working in the Barrio Adentro clinic. For her, the experience was dramatic enough to motivate a career change. Volunteers reported that only once they were engaged in health activism did they become conscious of the real need for such activism, which motivated them to continue.[10] Because they worked in the clinics and accompanied doctors on door-to-door censuses of the community's medical needs, volunteers witnessed the material benefits provided by Barrio Adentro as well as the challenges of poverty, homelessness, untreated medical conditions, and other social problems where they lived. By engaging in health activism, they began to hold a different view of their community and of themselves.

Grandparents Club Members

Participating in Grandparents Clubs also changed how people thought about themselves. The clubs transformed members' ideas about their bodies as stronger and more vital. Carla had been attending dance therapy classes for one month when she told me, "Look at me. Right now I feel very good. Very lively. I feel more agile. Before I didn't really know how to dance. Now that we're practicing, I like it a lot, I just dance and dance." This personal transformation was undeniably fun. Members did not describe physical activity in terms of sacrifice, pain, or hard work. It was not something they did when they would rather be doing something else. Quite the opposite: for these older adults, *bailoterapia* and other club activities produced high spirits and the satisfaction of moving one's body in purposeful activity.

Members came to view their participation in the Grandparents Club as essential for improving bodily health. When I met Inelda, she bragged to me that she had lost 9 kilos (approximately 20 pounds) since starting bailoterapia and changing her diet a few months earlier. She told me her knees did not hurt her as they once did and happily performed some leg squats as evidence. Participants relished dramatic stories about people who overcame paralysis of limbs through bailoterapia or people who started with the Grandparents Club using crutches but through the practice of dance therapy were able to walk and dance without assistance.[11]

Members associated club participation with the positive activation of mind and brain. Overall, socializing and exercising in public spaces were essential features of a shared cultural model of good health. Staying indoors was understood to lead to illness and even death. As one club member told me:

> On various occasions, I've told my family that I am truly very content [with the Grandparents Club], because this is what people like us have been missing, people of the third age.[12] . . . We should [still] go outside every day, right? Join in many activities. I believe that one just starts rusting inside the house . . . staying inside, staying inside, getting sick, getting fat, and worst of all, the brain is closing in on itself. Because being inside the house is just . . . every day you're dying a little more: not talking to anyone, not learning about anything, so the brain just goes to sleep . . . the mind closes.

Grandparents Clubs offered unique opportunities to socialize outdoors with other aging residents given the context of Caracas' *inseguridad,* the sense of insecurity and fear of crime that limited community life by prompting many to *encerrarse en la casa,* or lock themselves in," by 6:00 or 7:00 every evening. Having, as one woman called it, "a place to come to," where older adults could socialize and relax, was important. People frequently commented on the fact that before the institution of Grandparents Clubs no such spaces were available for older people from poor and working-class backgrounds.

Although club members did not claim that participation led to personal transformations as explicitly as community health workers did, conversations about their participation hinted at a changed sense of self. Eugenia, a lively seventy-eight-year-old member of one of Santa Teresa's Grandparents Clubs, differed from many club members. She was involved in many activities outside the home and always had a story to tell about something interesting she had done recently, like serving as an extra on the set of a telenovela. In addition to attending the Grandparents Club, she visited the local government day center for older adults and belonged to a dance group that performed choreographed dances in local theaters. She was one of the club members who signed up for free state-sponsored computer literacy classes for older adults offered by social work students in the neighborhood. Eugenia chose the name *cyberabuelita*, "little cyber-granny," for her email account and sent me email reports of her activities after I left Caracas. In an interview she described her experience of the Grandparents Club as a transformation of her personhood.

> AMY: Do you feel as if your health has improved?
>
> EUGENIA: Yes, yes, yes. Very much so, but more than anything, psychologically and emotionally. Because before I used to feel . . . left out, that I was nothing more than a slave in the home: cooking, washing, ironing, . . . with no incentive, without that something special that one needs, you know?
>
> AMY: And how have you changed?
>
> EUGENIA: I've changed a lot, because today I feel like a different person. For example, with [the Grandparents' Club] we go to the beach. Different people go, and we hang out like family. If we have to make a *sancocho* [traditional soup], each person helps to peel the potato, the yucca, the plantain, and cook it and serve it, and well . . . it's a beautiful brotherhood. Really great. . . . You know, we didn't have these before, these clubs for older adults.

Eugenia emphasized the sociality enjoyed through participation in the Grandparents Club. She referred to the spatial aspects of the change, associating interior home life with misery and isolation and outdoor activities with happiness and social connectedness. The difference was significant, leading her to feel like a different person.

Grandparents Clubs held political meanings for participants as well. They represented a substantive government benefit provided to older adults as part of the government's promise to reintegrate them into society. According to research participants and scholarly accounts, Venezuela's aging population suffered from neglect and even repression at the hands of previous governments. Neglect took the form of failure to provide retirement or other old-age pension payments and funding for social programs for older adults. Repression occurred at moments when aging Venezuelans took to the streets to demand their rights to government benefits. Older adults commonly protested what they described as the "misery" of a situation that became progressively worse when existing social benefits were cut during the late 1980s and 1990s. Elderly activists became notorious for their street protests involving powerful performances of deprivation and suffering, with protesters symbolically crucifying themselves, for example.[13] State authorities often responded with water cannons, rubber bullets, and tear gas.[14] Summarizing how past governments treated older adults, one Grandparents Club member told me, "Before, nobody paid any attention to the grandparents. . . . [U]p until recently grandparents were considered like, just trash."

When Grandparents Club members expressed excitement at having places to exercise, they were expressing pleasure about a change in how the Bolivarian government seemed to view them. During the early 2000s, the Chávez administration expanded medical care and social security for older adults and reorganized the National Institute of Geriatrics. These changes improved access to primary health care and led to a nearly 400 percent increase in the number of people receiving a state pension (from 387,000 in 1998 to more than 1.9 million in 2011).[15] The institute provided 600,000 new beneficiaries with economic and social services.[16] A 2009 study on old age and public policy conducted by the United Nations Economic Commission for Latin America and the Caribbean found that Venezuelan respondents were the most likely in the region to disagree that the state's treatment of the elderly was "bad or very bad," with over 60 percent of respondents claiming that treatment of the elderly was "good or very good."[17]

These survey findings corroborate claims made by research participants like Felicidad, who said:

> These benefits that we have now . . . I am sixty-nine years old and I've never seen such a thing, this is incredible! Whoever says it's not, they're not rational, truly they're not. . . . This is the best I've ever had. When have they ever taken us into account? I tell you that older persons have never been taken into account, no way, never. We now have therapies, we do exercises, we have Grandparents Clubs, in which I participate, we go on outings. I have even been to Cuba with my Grandparents Club.[18]

Estrella was a mild-mannered seventy-eight-year-old resident of Santa Teresa whose shuffling gait and slow speech belied a lucidity and mischievousness when she gossiped with club members. When a Cuban physical therapist was assigned to work with their club, Estrella began making sly jokes about which of the women should let the young handsome trainer live with them. In one of our conversations Estrella described the physical, psychological, and political significance of club participation.

> AMY: Has the Grandparents Club helped you?
>
> ESTRELLA: Yes, because if I don't go for a while I lay around in bed, and then at night I'm tossing and turning, but here I distract myself, you see? And when I go to sleep at night, before it was very difficult for me, but now I wake up feeling lighter on my feet . . . even though I don't do that much exercise here.
>
> AMY: Do you think the lives of older adults are improving now or is it similar to the way it has been before?
>
> ESTRELLA: No, now there are more [Grandparents] clubs.
>
> AMY: More clubs?
>
> ESTRELLA: Yes, more clubs. I see people of the third age as more optimistic now, because of these clubs and things . . .
>
> AMY: So who organizes and who funds these clubs?
>
> ESTRELLA: Well, this all started after Chávez. Before, people would have to pay to go to some therapy like this.
>
> AMY: So why did they fund these clubs for grandparents?
>
> ESTRELLA: Oh, I don't know, for our well-being, and because he [Chávez] is such a caring person and he loves the grandparents—you know that!

For Estrella, the very existence of these clubs served as a source of political satisfaction beyond the health benefits that membership provided. They represented a form of political recognition for older adults, indicating that they were now bodies who mattered to the state. Estrella scoffed at the fact that I would even ask why the government was offering these programs. In her mind it was obvious that this government cared about the well-being of its aging population.

HEALTH PROMOTION AS A MEANS OF COMMUNITY REVITALIZATION

Health Committees and Grandparents Clubs empowered members to participate in public life in ways that did not exist before. Engaging in health programs in public settings offered the pleasure of contributing to positive community change.

Community Health Workers' Census of Disabilities

Arriving an hour after the census's official start time, I was relieved to see others coming late to a plaza that was overflowing with people. At a glance it was obvious that a government-sponsored health event was under way. Half a dozen minibuses painted with the Libertador Municipality logo sat at the ready around the plaza's perimeter. Almost everyone was wearing a white doctor's coat or a red T-shirt bearing a Barrio Adentro logo or an uplifting revolutionary slogan. The plaza buzzed with the collective anticipation of two hundred doctors and community health workers preparing to do good work for the community.

I picked Lilian and Magdalena out of the crowd. They were engrossed in organizing teams to conduct a census of people with disabilities in Santa Teresa. The women paused their planning to introduce me to a handful of Cuban doctors and an administrator for the mayor's office of Libertador. The administrator was more interested in making conversation and cracking jokes than directing the event, and when I saw him later that day he greeted me from afar with a chirping, "Cooper! Cooper!" I noticed in the crowd other community health workers, including María and Carolina, whom I had known since my first visit in 2006. As the crowd started to coalesce into small groups, Lilian asked Carolina to stay with me so I was guaranteed a team to observe.

The census takers' impatience grew palpable as a lack of organizational hierarchy delayed their start. Community health workers, Cuban doctors, and municipal employees all wielded paperwork and clipboards. Some tried to match lists of street names with teams of census takers. Arguments erupted over which streets were covered and whether too many people were assigned to certain streets. A few groups decisively marched off while discussions continued, informally marking the start of the census. Amid the confusion Carolina followed a group entering a building across the street from the plaza and I trailed after her, unsure if we had begun the census.

The building's interior revealed a living situation attesting to community health workers' claims that this working-class neighborhood was home to more poverty than residents would admit. The space accommodated multiple families in conditions that officials would have classified as extreme poverty (*pobreza extrema*). The ground floor infrastructure was in disrepair. Ceilings and walls crumbled around a makeshift kitchen, with little food and a hodge-podge of gas ranges, and a common room was furnished with bare mattresses on the floor. Unsupervised children and toddlers played on the mattresses. At the back of the building sheets hung to demarcate private living spaces. I thought I detected expressions of shock on the faces of Carolina and other volunteers as we walked around. Community health workers directed the doctors to this building because they believed at least two people with disabilities lived there. Shortly after arriving, a pair of Cuban doctors identified someone they could assess for the census and disappeared behind a hanging sheet. Meanwhile, another doctor looked at our group with visible annoyance and said we didn't need to be there. He was right; most of our group was simply observing and taking up space. Adopting the doctor's tone of annoyance, a community health worker, María, ordered us to split up to get the census done faster.

The rest of the day Carolina and I accompanied a smaller group of doctors and activists on a preset route along an east-west corridor of the neighborhood. The Cuban doctors seemed unbothered that the housing we encountered, mostly multistory apartment blocks fronted by locked doors with thick metal bars, restricted their access to households. A member of our group would yell past the bars to get a resident to open the door. Sometimes residents responded by calling out their windows or coming onto balconies. One of the doctors had a small pad of paper on which she noted the names of buildings where nobody answered, as well as the names of the few people we encountered who had suspected disabilities. Later we met a doctor from a different group of census takers who said they found only two people with untreated disabilities on their route. Although we might assume doctors and activists would express relief at a low demand for disability services, they seemed ambivalent about the census outcome, as if they hoped to find more people who needed their help. I knew that community health workers as well as Cuban doctors here assessed the success of their labor in terms of identifying and resolving unmet medical needs.

The census was more than an opportunity for community health workers to do good works; it was a way for them to enjoy embodying their role. They believed their work was essential to improving population health and reversing a history of social exclusion. Knowing they were doing this was a source of deep satisfaction. This was evidenced in the way people talked about their work. The day before the census, I accompanied María to a Barrio Adentro diagnostic center at the new Bolivarian University, and as we chatted with one of the directors, María mentioned the upcoming census. The director exclaimed, "Oh! It really moves me to hear that you'll be doing this; before people were hidden away and it's so important to help them." Visibly pleased with the praise, María responded that it was time to end the stigma associated with having a disability. On census day, my conversations with Carolina invoked the value of volunteer work. Trailing behind our Cuban doctors, Carolina explained that even after five years of having Barrio Adentro clinics, many people in Santa Teresa still did not believe the Cubans were actual doctors. Encoded in this statement was a claim about the importance of community health workers like herself. Given doctors' liminal and sometimes contested presence, community health workers served as liaisons between doctors and local residents. The main functions of community health workers in the census were to show support for the government's work and to liaise with local residents who might hesitate to accept offers of help. They vouched for the legitimacy of the doctors and if necessary deflected criticism and organized protection from physical threats of violence from right-wing opposition residents.

Doing this work was satisfying, and doing it in public space lent a special satisfaction. Public events allowed community health workers to take pleasure in visibly collaborating on projects they viewed as revitalizing their communities. An important aspect of their participation was the clothing activists wore. Volunteers identified themselves through their clothing choices, often advertising their support for the Chávez government. Barrio Adentro provided red and gray shirts identifying the wearer as a Health Committee member, but activists had other options also. Red T-shirts were the most common choice. Members also wore red hats and T-shirts with the slogans of other government programs, Chávez himself, or the socialist party, PSUV (fig. 14).[19] During my fieldwork, I amassed a substantial collection of hats and T-shirts from community health workers who assumed that I would similarly enjoy identifying with these causes. The day of the census, passersby who supported the government's social programs noticed our attire and started conversations to learn what we were doing and to share a moment of solidarity. Community health workers' clothes also drew attention from residents who opposed the government. One passerby yelled at the activists in our group, calling them *chavistas* in a dismissive tone. Without missing a beat, one of our group, a stylish man in his early twenties, called back that we were doing community work (*trabajo comunitario*), providing health care. The resident's attempt to disparage the group backfired by offering volunteers an

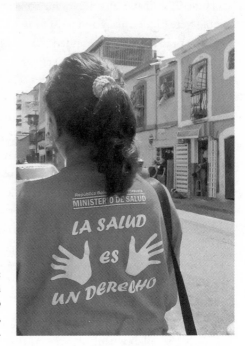

FIGURE 14. "Health is a right": A community health worker in Santa Teresa turns around to make a point during a conversation, 2006. Photo by the author.

opening to publicly articulate their virtuousness. In this way, both positive and negative attention from local residents reinforced volunteers' sense of moral and political certitude.

Grandparents Clubs in Public Space

Although both of Santa Teresa's Grandparents Clubs held exercise classes in schoolyards with guards who restricted access to the general public, their members socialized, exercised, and performed in various public spaces. Club leaders organized field trips and public performances that allowed members to enjoy a visibility that produced a sense of belonging and empowerment.

I accompanied club members on one of their outings on an uncharacteristically chilly day in March, traveling by Metro to a meet-and-greet in a public park. Even the journey between Santa Teresa and Parque del Oeste in the western zone of the city offered opportunities for club members to embody public personas as vibrant and engaged citizens. After congregating in the neighborhood's central plaza we walked as a group to the Metro station.

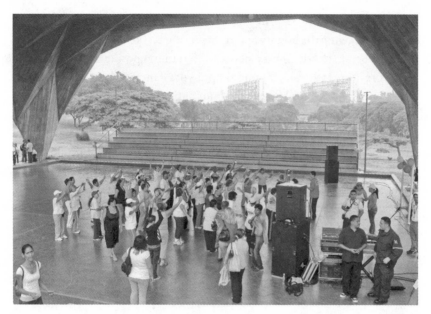

FIGURE 15. Grandparents Club meet-up in eastern Caracas, 2009. Photo by the author.

Everybody wore baby-blue T-shirts identifying the club in large block letters. The group—all older women—joked around as we neared the station, then took turns stepping in front of a long line in the Metro to claim their free tickets (an often remarked upon government benefit for older adults). Boisterous conversation continued as the train passed station after station aboveground and we arrived at the hundred-acre park, leaving the commotion of commuters and street vendors behind.

Rushing toward a concrete domed sports pitch to avoid drizzles of rain, we joined about a hundred people from Grandparents Clubs across the municipality for a morning of dancing and socializing. The other groups (comprising mostly older women) wore matching clothing, too. One club sported pink velvet outfits and visors. Another group wore T-shirts that joyfully proclaimed, "Revolutionize yourself with physical activity!" Two hip DJs manned the sound system, playing booming chart hits to match the energy of the crowd. People's grandchildren milled about while club members socialized with Cuban sports trainers from different neighborhoods. Soon an enormous bailoterapia session got under way (fig. 15). When people stopped to take a break, officials from the municipal government passed out snacks. Each person received an apple, a pear, a plum, and an apricot neatly arranged on a Styrofoam plate and wrapped in cling film. People sat on the bleachers enjoying the bounty and commenting on how nice the fruit tasted. After the break, club members spent fifteen minutes posing for group photos before breaking into pairs for impromptu salsa dancing.

Grandparents Clubs blurred the boundaries of activities that promoted fun and activities that promoted health. Throughout the festive event, participants laughed and joked among themselves. They displayed none of the seriousness or focused attention on the body we associate with people enacting exercise regimes. Nobody attended or danced out of a sense of duty or guilt. Such events boosted participants' identities as active and publicly engaged older adults, implicitly challenging stereotypes of older adults as frail and socially isolated.

I conducted fieldwork at various public events recognizing the vitality of aging Venezuelans. One of these was a celebration of the Día del Adulto Mayor, a national day for older adults held in the city's politically charged Plaza Bolívar. Members of Santa Teresa's Grandparents Club performed a choreographed dance for the event and received certificates and medals commending their participation (which they showed off at the club's bailoterapia class later that day, hamming it up for photos). Official speeches honored "the country's grandparents," described how the revolutionary government was improving their lives, and called for further improvements. One speaker declared, "We have to find a holistic solution for the nutritional needs of older adults. We have the political will. Our president said we have to dignify older adults!" Another speaker acknowledged Chávez's humanity for addressing the needs of people who were "least recognized" in society but noted that the work was not nearly completed. She got a round of applause when she announced, "We must demand social justice for older adults!"

Some public events manifestly empowered older adults in Grandparents Clubs by encouraging them to speak for themselves. One was an annual pageant to select Santa Teresa's King and Queen of the Third Age. Winners represented the neighborhood in a citywide pageant whose prize was riding the Carnaval float that year. Almost every entrant was a member of a local Grandparents Club. Women wore formal gowns and heels, some showing off flamboyant matching Carnaval headdresses; men wore suits (fig. 16). The club's organizer, Lilian, arranged for a stage, a sound system, and chairs to be set up in the neighborhood's main plaza.

The competition included a question and answer session in which contestants offered "advice for the younger generation." Statements ranged from

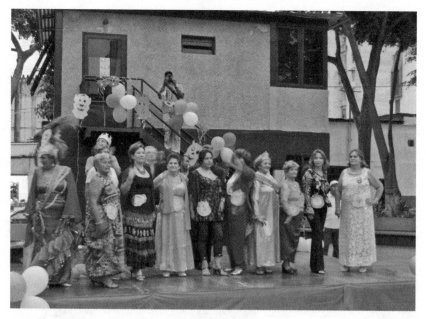

FIGURE 16. Pageant for the King and Queen of the Third Age, 2009. Photo by the author.

generic advice to politically and historically situated commentaries. Contestants' voices reverberated off the concrete apartment buildings that flanked the plaza as they took turns speaking into the microphone. They made declarations: "People must have morals and take responsibility for their lives!" "Let's keep struggling and overcome!" (¡Vamos luchando y vencer!); "Smile at life. Life is beautiful!" "Educate yourselves, study, do a lot of sports, don't take drugs!"; "Young ones! Don't leave the *abuelas* [grandmothers] in the home when you go out. Take them with you!" The audience of family members, friends, and neighbors applauded after each person spoke. Contestants seemed to enjoy this opportunity to publicly address their neighbors and share their worldviews and basked in the attention. The eventual winner, Eugenia, beamed throughout, standing proudly with one leg positioned in front of the other like a coquettish beauty pageant participant. The event promoted a counternarrative to accepted ideas about the elderly, as the men and women revealed themselves as engaged citizens with active, vital bodies.

The activities club members performed and the identities they embodied in public spaces altered the meanings of these public spaces, even if temporarily (fig. 17). Staging a celebration of aging residents' vitality in a relatively

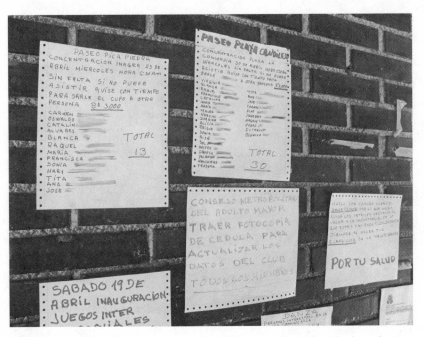

FIGURE 17. Flyers announcing Grandparents Club outings, 2008. Photo by the author.

derelict and "unsafe" plaza resignified that space as one capable of promoting pro-social causes for the benefit of the community.

THE MEANING OF PARTICIPATION

The word *participation* (*participación*) held special meaning for both community health workers and club members. It has the same meaning in Spanish and English, but in Bolivarian Venezuela the notion of participation carried an extra political significance due to the government's emphasis on popular participation (*participación popular*) as a means of empowerment and social change. The 1999 Constitution redefined Venezuela's political system as a participatory democracy, meaning that ordinary people were encouraged and expected to play direct roles in community, regional, and national government.[20] Popular participation became a core principle of political action in Bolivarian Venezuela.

Using terms like popular power (*poder popular*) and popular participation, state officials called on historically marginalized groups (the poor, working classes, women, indigenous groups, Afro-Venezuelans) to organize themselves and engage in the work of government, mostly at the local level. This call to participation invoked an older government discourse about Venezuelans as the rightful owners of the nation's oil wealth, revived in the Chávez era with slogans like "Ahora es de todos" (Now it [the nation-state] belongs to us all). Participatory discourse encouraged Venezuelans to not just take the goods and services that the government provided, but organize and make demands on the state and shape government administration. During this period massive numbers of Venezuelans, most of them poor or working class, became decision makers and service providers in government programs promoting health, education, housing, community governance, and land and water rights.[21]

Official narratives aimed at community health workers and Grandparents Club members emphasized the transformative potential of participación. In a Ministry of Health pamphlet explaining how to form a Grandparents Club, a third of the text was devoted to answering the question, "What is participation?" The answer read in part:

> Participation is a form of social intervention that allows individuals to recognize each other as agents with a shared identity based on common interests, expectations, and demands, who are able to translate these into autonomous collective action.

The pamphlet included pronouncements such as "Participation is a right established by our Constitution"; "Participation is a right of citizenship"; "Participating in Grandparents Clubs means improving your quality of life"; and "Onward toward the exercise of citizens' power."[22] The pamphlet made it patently clear that Grandparents Clubs were not merely places to exercise.

Research participants also referred to participation as a special transformative practice. To "participate" in government-sponsored health promotion activities did not mean merely improving one's health; it meant seizing an opportunity to transform society. Community health worker, Mariángela, explained her entrée into health promotion:

> Before Chávez I was "nonparticipatory": I did not participate. I dedicated myself to my house, to my work, to my son, to my husband. But there wasn't this opportunity before, there was nothing to stimulate you. Presidents came and went, they did their own health fairs using their personnel from government institutions. But to give participation to the pueblo, to let you be the protagonist of your own destiny, so you could be the one who helps to solve problems? This is thanks to the president because this national project involves the inclusion of the excluded.

Since beginning community health work, Mariángela viewed herself in a different light, as a "participatory" person—an activist who worked for the greater good. I believed her. Through her physical presence and speech, Mariángela embodied her narrative of empowerment via participation. She exuded self-confidence and a sense of righteousness about community health work. She was one of the only people I knew in Santa Teresa who spoke openly about her role in building socialism (others tended to speak euphemistically, probably to lessen the potential for controversy in the politically polarized neighborhood).

Research participants portrayed participation in health promotion programs as a moral and political imperative. A man in his sixties named Octavio attended the Grandparents Club where I spent the most time observing. One day he visited when the club was hosting a party to celebrate the birthdays of members born that month. Carving out a moment to address the group while they distributed pieces of syrupy cake, Octavio gave an impromptu speech. He recently began volunteering in a nearby municipal office for older adults and advised club members to sign up for activities and field trips there. "You need to *demand* your rights as older adults," he told them. "Your club here is very new, it's only been around for a few months, but you will grow stronger." He ended with the exhortation, "It's not enough to simply *attend* an event. You must *participate*!"

I see a parallel between community health workers and Grandparents Club members discussing the imperative to *participar* in health promotion and patients urging each other to *aprovechar*, or take advantage of, government medicine (discussed in chap. 4). Engaging with health programs offered political benefits beyond health care access by offering individuals a sense of being someone who mattered to the state. Whether *participando* or *aprovechando*, people who long felt abandoned by the state and excluded from public life took pleasure in the feeling of being taken into account. Participación and aprovechando were different, though: participation implied a form of social action that went beyond seeking health in an individualized sense. Participation demanded collaboration with other likeminded people, often in public spaces, and promised to revitalize communities as well as individual bodies.

Community health workers and Grandparents Club members idealized participation in government health promotion programs. The fact that participation promised remarkable benefits helps explain the pleasure many people expressed when engaging in these programs. Unsurprisingly,

Bolivarian social programs established high expectations for personal and social change that they could not always meet. We might hypothesize that the more a social program promised, the greater the disappointment and displeasure when expectations went unmet. The next chapter examines community participation in another health promotion program, a government mission to rehabilitate people who were homeless and addicted to drugs or alcohol. This program elicited displeasure from neighborhood volunteers for not working as expected. Analyzing the reasons for this displeasure reveals even more about the social and political significance of health care in Bolivarian Venezuela.

SIX

The Limits of Citizenship

AS MORE REASONABLE PEOPLE TOOK REFUGE from the muggy midday heat, I struggled to match Lilian's purposeful stride along the streets near her house. In clipped Caraqueño Spanish, she delivered a rapid-fire monologue about new government programs in the neighborhood. The indefatigable health activist pointed out abandoned buildings that she hoped they would acquire and put to use—for example, as a *casa de alimentación*, or soup kitchen. Rounding a corner, we nearly tripped over a man sleeping on flattened cardboard boxes (fig. 18). Lilian gestured in his direction with pursed lips (a movement akin to pointing) and said, "See him? We are going to help all these people, the *indigentes* [indigents]. So they're not living on the street."

This was one of many promises Lilian made that day in 2006. She held an unfailingly optimistic view of what members of a community could accomplish through grit and collaboration with Bolivarian government officials. I wondered what Lilian imagined community members could do to help people who lived on the street. I had recently completed participant observation in Chicago among homeless women and was struck by the intractable forces that could make homelessness a permanent condition. Lilian was hopeful. She had just begun volunteering in a government social program rehabilitating people who lived on the streets—the city's so-called indigents. The program was only a few months old, and community activists had begun training that summer.

I recalled that conversation when, three years later, Lilian denigrated the indigentes she formerly promised to help. In 2009 she urged me to join her at a grand opening for a senior citizens' center in a formerly abandoned building. Lilian explained that the building had become an *invasión*, or squat, inhabited by "locos y indigentes"—crazies and indigents. She cheerfully

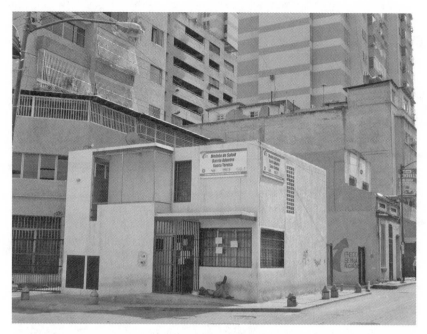

FIGURE 18. Man sleeping in the shade of a Barrio Adentro clinic, 2008. Photo by the author.

reported that community activists and government workers had transformed the site into an inclusive and peaceful center where older adults could socialize and take classes. Lilian talked effusively about the building's new purpose. She did not comment on the irony of the fact that squatters were forced to the streets by a social welfare project helping a different class of vulnerable persons. Lilian's apparent disinterest in the well-being of homeless people was in sharp contrast to her attitude in 2006. I wondered what had changed.

I observed as community health activists experienced homeless outreach first as a source of pleasure, then as a source of displeasure. In 2006, residents of Santa Teresa enthusiastically joined a government rehabilitation program to help the homeless, but within a short time the program lost community support and volunteers began considering it a failure. Volunteer health activists embarked on outreach with gusto but ended up marginalizing the already marginalized urban homeless after their work failed to swiftly recuperate them.

My research revealed that indigentes evoked displeasure among well-meaning activists because they threatened a logic of health and healing that undergirded Bolivarian social programs. The government's Negra Hipólita mission portrayed indigentes as the prime example of social marginalization who would be healed and empowered by participating in the program. Successfully rehabilitating this population would highlight the success of a participatory politics of demarginalization and citizenship. However, failure to enlist people in this government-sponsored process of transformation threatened the idea that people would embrace opportunities to empower themselves if given the chance. Analyzing volunteers' displeasure with indigentes for failing to demarginalize themselves reveals that even a joyful politics of inclusionary health care has limits and unintended consequences for certain social groups.

POPULAR AND MEDIA REPRESENTATIONS
OF INDIGENTES

Venezuelans understood indigentes to be people who were literally living on the streets (or in parks or plazas) and addicted to drugs or alcohol. The association between street homelessness and addiction seemed fairly accurate. According to the president of a public foundation for addiction treatment in Caracas, 90 percent of people living on the streets in Venezuela were addicted to drugs or alcohol and approximately 10 percent suffered from a serious mental illness such as schizophrenia or bipolar disorder.[1]

Street homelessness in Caracas resulted from a number of large-scale social problems such as poverty, lack of affordable housing, substance use, and mental illness coalescing in individual bodies. Homelessness was a major concern in Caracas, and indigentes comprised just a small minority of the population of *personas sin techo* (lit., "people without a roof"). Rapid urbanization during the twentieth century meant that new arrivals often built housing into hillside barrios at the periphery of the formal city. Subsequent arrivals built up, adding stories to the self-constructed architecture. By the early 2000s most city residents felt there was nowhere left to build. In spite of constitutional guarantees of "dignified housing" and state promises to build housing for personas sin techo, the rate of construction had not alleviated the problem. This pervasive housing shortage prompted large numbers of homeless people to squat in disused buildings across the city, sometimes as an orchestrated act of protest but more often as a survival strategy when faced with no other viable options. Amid this housing crisis, people identified as indigentes were the most vulnerable and marginalized of the hundreds of thousands of people who did not have a place to call home. Yet they were also seen to be the population most responsible for their situation and most likely to cause problems for other neighborhood residents.

Santa Teresa's residents described the neighborhood's biggest problems as ones that they directly linked to *indigencia* (indigence). Residents told me the parish's biggest problems were crime, violence, alcoholism, drug abuse, prostitution, indigentes, trash, and community apathy. When I asked Roberto, a teacher who worked at a Jesuit primary school in a nearby barrio, how Santa Teresa compared to other parts of Caracas he quickly responded that it was full of indigentes and dangerous. As we walked through the neighborhood he led me on a detour around the parish's central plaza, noting that it was very unsafe. When residents spoke about the threat of violence in the neighborhood they focused on the plaza as a site of danger. The few times I heard stories about murders in the neighborhood, most were said to have taken place in this plaza.[2] The plaza also was where one was most likely to see disheveled people drinking alcohol and sleeping in public—people whom residents identified as indigentes. Although criminal activities were not viewed as the sole purview of indigentes, popular discourse consistently associated them with criminality.

Beliefs about the causes of indigencia existed in tension with each other. Many residents of Santa Teresa viewed indigentes as caught in a web of historical and structural forces that were difficult to transcend. At the same time, they asserted the role of individual agency in self-improvement, particularly in cases of substance use. A Barrio Adentro user and Santa Teresa resident named Carmen said of the people treated by the Negra Hipólita program:

> The thing is, this is an addiction, a very serious illness and people have to become aware of it and really want to live . . . for [some]one to leave all these things behind one has to gain awareness. Alcohol totally destroys you, drugs . . . all of this destroys you . . . it's a question of awareness.

The news media vacillated between representing indigentes as victims and as harbingers of criminality and filth. This inconsistent portrayal drew on contradictory understandings of indigentes as subject to structural forces outside their control, on the one hand, and as personally responsible for their problems, on the other. For example, a four-page feature story in a national newspaper depicted indigentes as victims of unscrupulous scrap collectors. The journalist described a widespread urban problem in which scrap metal collectors provided indigentes with tools and encouraged them to steal metal from public art, bridges, and utility lines, which they exchanged for drugs.[3] The article included photos and personal stories of indigentes who struggled with addiction and exploitation at the hands of scrappers. It featured a former minister in charge of the Negra Hipólita mission who accused scrappers of inducing drug addiction and exploiting indigentes for profit. The minister bemoaned the fact that "contraband traders incite the poorest people in Caracas to rob."[4] Here we see an awareness that people defined as indigentes were vulnerable and mistreated.

However, most media reports cast indigentes as criminals, not victims. An article in the same newspaper, titled "Indigentes Up to Their Old Tricks," included photos of a derelict public plaza strewn with trash and two people sleeping against a curb, with a byline claiming, "They sleep in the trash, generate scandals, and engage in unseemly acts."[5] The story was billed as a report on the Negra Hipólita mission's recruiting of indigentes along the edge of Santa Teresa's western border, but most of the copy space was dedicated to criticizing the filth and immorality of indigentes. The journalist wrote, "Four indigentes slept in the middle of the day, recovering from the night before.... [T]hey were immersed in trash and surrounded by liquor bottles."[6]

Negative media characterizations of indigentes reflected broader debates over the use of public space in Venezuela under Chávez. Officials invested heavily in programs to recuperate (*recuperar*) public spaces that held historical and cultural significance. Urban recuperation focused on the *casco histórico,* the colonial city center that included Santa Teresa. According to popular opinion, these spaces had deteriorated over time because the state and private citizens neglected them. Many sites were deemed dangerous, dysfunctional, and aesthetically compromised. Recuperation projects proved highly controversial: residents and officials often clashed with indigentes and informal street vendors (*buhoneros*) targeted for removal from such spaces.

Recuperation efforts framed indigentes (and buhoneros) as undermining the proper use of public space. A 2008 news story described neighborhood councils whose members partnered with the mayor's office to revitalize a pedestrian boulevard, Paseo Anauco. The author wrote that council members "wanted to convert it into a tourist space for the enjoyment of Caraqueños."[7] A major impediment to their plan was "the indigentes who prowled the zone, who continually carry large amounts of trash and leave it strewn around, and who bust water pipes in order to collect drinking water, bathe, and wash their clothes."[8] The story included a photo of a person "prowling" near a bridge on the boulevard, a disheveled older woman wearing a nightgown. It suggested that forced removal of indigentes was an inevitable part of recuperating the boulevard. In other words, improving community public spaces seemed to involve denying access to people viewed as less deserving of access to them. Public space revitalization efforts concerned with order, safety, and cleanliness paralleled concerns of earlier eras of governance in Latin America. Portrayals of indigentes as a threat to public order resonated with positivist hygienic discourses common in the early twentieth century that explicitly contrasted social groups in terms of civilized and barbaric tendencies.

In contrast to urban renewal efforts that figured indigentes as a problem to be removed or excluded, the Negra Hipólita mission focused on improving the lives of the indigentes. Officials described the Negra Hipólita project as revolutionary in its promise to usher in new forms of dignity and social integration for an especially marginalized population.

THE NEGRA HIPÓLITA MISSION

On Christmas Eve 2005 the revolutionary government announced a social welfare program called Misión Negra Hipólita to "aid at-risk groups including the homeless, extremely poor, or drug-addicted people."[9] The program would offer housing and medical, social, and vocational services to people living on the streets. According to the minister in charge, "The new mission would be based primarily on direct community action against the problems of vulnerable groups."[10] The government called on local residents to volunteer as the first point of contact in recruiting indigentes to participate. Discussing the new mission on his television show, *Aló Presidente,* in 2006, Chávez said, "It is a very Christian, very humanitarian mission."[11]

La Negra Hipólita (Black Hipólita) was an actual historical figure with immense symbolic resonance. Hipólita Bolívar was an Afro-Venezuelan slave who lived in the late 1700s. At age twenty she served as wet nurse to Simón Bolívar, who became a key figure in Latin America's struggle for independence from Spain. Known across the region as el Libertador (the Liberator), he is also revered as the founding father of the Venezuelan nation-state. Bolívar freed his family's slaves in 1821, including Hipólita, whom he claimed to love as a family member. Given Bolívar's pervasive identification with an independent Venezuela, Hipólita personifies a nurturing figure not only for Bolívar but also for the Venezuelan nation-state.

The Chávez government drew on the symbolism of this nurturing mother figure by portraying the mission as a humanistic welfare project to rehabilitate persons who had lost the ability to care for themselves. The program subverted the historical reality of Hipólita as caregiver to the elite and wealthy of Venezuela. As namesake for the Negra Hipólita mission, Hipólita's powers of nurturance and mothering focused on the most impoverished and marginalized people in society. The minister originally charged with implementing the social mission explained, "Negra Hipólita represents love and the generosity of Venezuelan mothers, equality, solidarity, and justice for a neglected Venezuelan group who are filled with misery."[12]

The program portrayed indigentes as able to heal and reintegrate into society even after years of living on the street. In the idealized process of rehabilitation indigentes received encouragement from community volunteers, participated in the Negra Hipólita program, and enjoyed social reinclusion. The ultimate goal of the mission was to enact social justice. The program built on assumptions about health that undergirded other Chávez-era social programs, advocating for empowerment via demarginalization. It challenged popular assumptions about indigentes as undesirables who ruined public spaces by their very presence. In this model of government intervention, community revitalization could only occur alongside a rehabilitation process that dignified people living on the streets.

ROMANTICIZING COMMUNITY WORK

It was impossible to ignore the pleasure Santa Teresa residents took in the Negra Hipolita mission in the summer of 2006 when they began training. Trainee volunteers attended a number of meetings, including a multiday training course specifically for their community at the headquarters of the Ministry for Popular Participation and Social Development (MINPADES). Volunteers found discourses of inclusion, popular participation, and empowerment compelling and motivating. Before attempting to implement their training in actual interactions with indigentes, volunteers and some state workers tended to idealize the mission's work and the rehabilitation process that participants were meant to undergo.

Program volunteers and employees romanticized the treatment experience and the role the community would play in rehabilitation. At one neighborhood meeting, volunteers and I sat at tiny desks in an elementary school classroom. While participants engaged in a heated debate over whether they needed government identification cards to denote their status as Negra Hipólita volunteers (evidence of a wider cultural concern about identity documents and authentication of oneself in a city where everyday purchases of snacks or school supplies required one's *cédula,* or national identity card), I struck up a conversation with Elisabela, a woman in her fifties sitting behind me. She was eager to talk to me about the new mission—how much it was needed, what it would do, and who it would help. She told me with bright eyes about the refuges (*refugios*) where people went for therapy. She saw one of the rehabilitation centers on television. She said they got healthy food, lived in the mountains, and got a psychologist and a psychiatrist, and when they returned they got money to help them settle down and work.

In Elisabela's narrative, the rehabilitation center sounded like a vacation complex, an escape from the harsh realities of daily life in Caracas. The treatment process sounded smooth and unproblematic. From Elisabela's vague description, it was not clear what rehabilitation would actually look like or what kinds of activities people would participate in while they lived at the center, not to mention the fact that much of the discourse around the mission idealized community-based rehabilitation, which did not mesh with her description of the mountain refuge. She described the end goal of reintegration into the community as a matter of fact rather than as a contingency among various possible outcomes. I wondered what kind of sustainable work she imagined people would find upon their return to a city with high levels of unemployment and labor informality.

Training sessions humanized the figure of the indigente and elicited spontaneous expressions of emotion from volunteer trainees. Later that summer, I attended a full day and evening of a Negra Hipólita training course for Santa Teresa residents who wanted to volunteer. Government employees who ran these courses for volunteers from all over Caracas facilitated participatory discussions that focused not only on the logistics of recruiting and rehabilitating indigentes in the social mission but also on the proper way to think about indigentes, the personal struggles of volunteers, and the radical potential of participatory democracy.

Facilitators portrayed indigentes as agentive individuals subject to histories of marginalization. One facilitator told the group, "Some people think the Negra Hipólita mission is to take this 'trash' off the street and hide it away, put it away. No. We help them from the streets so they'll be subjects, not objects, which is what they are now." Later that day, a different facilitator picked up on this theme. He said to volunteers, "We're not saying 'poor indigent.' They are not *pobrecitos* [poor little things]. Rather, [we ask], how are we to resolve extreme misery in our community?" In their attempts to humanize indigentes, facilitators tried to delegitimize pervasive stereotypes of indigentes as either morally corrupt or helpless victims. State employees urged volunteers to recognize and treat indigentes as subjects, as human beings like all others.

Facilitators encouraged volunteers to engage emotionally in the day's discussions by suggesting that their personal struggles resonated with the challenges indigentes faced. One government employee pointed out that most of the volunteers in the room were women and that women were both victims of and participants in a pernicious culture of machismo. She noted that many of the volunteers were disadvantaged because they had been raised in single-parent households and were single parents themselves. By pointing out structural difficulties that affected many of Santa Teresa's volunteers, facilitators emphasized the fact that people's lives are shaped by forces outside their personal control. State employees encouraged volunteers to embrace empathy and self-reflection when working with indigentes. "The first process of therapy is giving love to people," claimed a facilitator.

State employees told volunteers that rehabilitating indigentes helped enact participatory democracy and social justice. One facilitator reminded volunteers that the work of Negra Hipólita was connected to the struggles for collective ownership of political power. "How can we begin to feel like the rightful owners of Venezuela? *¡Es nuestro!* [It belongs to us!]," she exclaimed. She reminded volunteers, "This revolution will not be easy. The past eight years have not been easy," suggesting that transforming society to end social inequalities would entail hard work. Throughout, the goal of recruiting and rehabilitating indigentes was linked discursively to the personal experiences and emotions of individual volunteers and discussed as part of a larger national project of social change that was, without doubt, moving forward.

The volunteers' responses to the training suggested that they found it energizing and cathartic. In one activity, volunteers sat in a circle recounting personal hardships that made them want to join the mission's work. A middle-aged man named Rodolfo stood up and shared his life story, revealing that he was a *niño de la calle* (homeless street kid). He suffered sexual abuse as a child and became an alcoholic. He said he overcame these problems and was now eager to help others living with the same problems. At the end of the day the group stood in a circle and sang a song while holding hands. Each person stated how the training had helped him or her. Many choked up when it was their turn to talk. Afterward, participants walked around the room hugging each other and crying.

Engaging in the Negra Hipólita mission allowed people who experienced varying degrees of impoverishment and social exclusion to feel a sense of empowerment by helping others. Volunteers would have experienced deprivations or discrimination of some form during their lives. Many benefited from Chávez-era social programs like Barrio Adentro. Santa Teresa's volunteers took pleasure in the idea that they could help a group of people who seemed demonstrably more marginal than they were. Doing this work was a way to enact their own inclusion and citizenship by bringing other marginalized people into the fold of government social welfare and self-directed empowerment. Volunteers also hoped this work would revitalize their community by ending street homelessness and its associated concerns.

These early meetings instilled in volunteers an unproblematic understanding of the rehabilitation process. People seemed to assume the program would enjoy success, just as Lilian breezily promised that Santa Teresa would eliminate homelessness that day we passed the man sleeping in the doorway. The figure of the marginal indigente became an emotionally charged focus for government promises of radical social change. However, when volunteers began to engage with the indigentes in Santa Teresa, certain realities eroded their idealized vision of rehabilitation.

INTRANSIGENT ILLNESSES, UNSUITABLE CITIZENS

As soon as volunteers began outreach work, their anticipatory pleasure over rehabilitating indigentes gave way to frustration and confusion. I noticed the change later that summer when I attended a meeting between the neighborhood's Negra Hipólita volunteers and staff. The group met in a shiny new ministry building thirty minutes from Santa Teresa by Metro. More than two dozen volunteers crammed into a well-appointed conference room with picture windows overlooking the hills. Most attendees were the same people who went to the all-day training session. Yet this meeting's tone differed from that high-spirited training session. Volunteers had found the work much harder than they had imagined. They came to the meeting full of questions.

Every volunteer who spoke had a story about someone she was trying to help, and in every case it was not working. There seemed to be two types of problems. In some cases, volunteers received agreement from indigentes to seek help but then did not know what to do. They literally did not know where to take the individual or whom to contact to pick him or her up. One woman said she was trying to help a man who lives on the streets, is an alcoholic, and smokes six packs of cigarettes per day. She told the group that she had all his information. Now what should she do? These logistical issues related to lack of coordination between the Negra Hipólita staff and neighborhood volunteers. It seemed that the program got off the ground before facilities were in place near Santa Teresa to process participants. Some facilities also reached capacity, and program staff had to find alternative rehabilitation sites.

More volunteers complained of a second problem, the unwillingness of indigentes to accept their offers of help. One woman told the group, "There's a woman who came to me. She has a son who's using drugs, and she wants him to go to rehabilitation." A volunteer interrupted her, correctly guessing what she was going to say next. "But he doesn't want help? That's the problem, isn't it?," she asked rhetorically. A middle-aged woman with crimson-dyed hair (a beauty practice that communicated affinity with *chavismo*) asked how to help an "entirely alcoholic family" living together in an apartment. "The mother and two children are alcoholic and don't want help," she said. Rodolfo, the man who talked about having been a homeless street kid at the previous week's meeting, complained that he had been trying to recruit a homeless boy into the rehabilitation program, but the boy kept "using him" by asking for coffees and other things and Rodolfo did not know what to do.

A facilitator named Miguel told a story to illustrate the intransigent nature of homelessness. He said a group of people was living on the street near the ministry building in the upper-middle-class suburb where they were meeting that day. The group based themselves near some stairs that led to a viaduct, with a bed and jerry-rigged electrical access that powered a television. He explained, "We are convincing them, little by little, to come with us for help." A volunteer cried out in frustration, "I thought we were going to be taking them away!" Miguel replied, "Yes, but we can't take them by force.

Don't believe this is easy." As in the United States, authorities in Venezuela could not treat people with substance abuse problems or another psychiatric illness against their will unless they represented a threat of harm to themselves or to others. The woman's exclamation expressed the frustration many of the volunteers felt about what they thought would be a straightforward process. Her statement evoked ideas that state employees tried to avoid, that the rehabilitation program was the human equivalent of taking trash off the street and out of public view.

A clinical psychologist named Oswaldo led the second half of the meeting, trying to recalibrate volunteers' expectations. In a smooth authoritative voice he reminded the group that they were fighting extreme poverty and social exclusion. He described the people they wanted to help as "people in maximum exclusion" and emphasized that "the fundamental goal is social reinsertion." Oswaldo explained this was a political issue because social exclusion was a "fundamental feature of capitalism." His narrative mirrored what the other facilitators told volunteers in training, that homelessness and drug addiction were structural problems of poverty and that the work of the Negra Hipólita mission was tied to larger struggles at the national level to transform society.

Oswaldo broke from the program's official discourse when he acknowledged the pervasive impediments facing indigentes. He admitted, "In reality, there are some people who cannot be rehabilitated. I know the president wants to get everyone off the street. I agree. But it's just not that easy." Oswaldo's matter-of-fact acknowledgment that rehabilitation for people living on the streets was often incomplete reflected what medical researchers, clinicians, and anthropologists have observed about homelessness,[13] but it did not assuage volunteers' frustrations. For volunteers, people who refused state services were not just doing their bodies a disservice; they were rejecting a moral obligation to empower themselves when the opportunity presented itself.

Even people who did sign up for rehabilitation could evoke discontent in the eyes of community members. In the nearby barrio 23 de Enero, health activist Clara led the effort to institute a Negra Hipólita rehabilitation facility close to her home. Neighborhood residents complained about the unsuitability of the facility's location, citing problems caused by indigentes who lived there. The community's reaction led the government to shut down the facility and move rehabilitation services outside the city. When I asked Clara to explain what happened she empathized with the residents.

There was a [Negra Hipólita] rehabilitation center here, but the entire community started coming to me, to complain. . . .

You know what [the indigentes] are like, they come disrobed, wounded, cut up, with knives, with guns! They had been causing a grave problem of crime and health. They bathed nude out there, as the building was next to a stream, they took the opportunity to bathe, and little children could witness this spectacle. . . .

Sure, of course they are the priority [for getting social services], but not here, inside a sector [neighborhood], because it generates problems.

Residents also complained that indigentes visited the communal soup kitchens that served other people in the neighborhood. Clara defended their complaints, stating they represented a health threat.

[Indigents] are from the street [*son de la calle*], they carry many diseases, and it's undesirable, because [they can carry] the virus for tuberculosis. . . . They [carry] strong flus and, well, infections that they can transmit through their hands, you know.

When describing indigentes as "from the street," Clara used the permanent verb form *ser* (to be; "son de la calle"), suggesting that the indigentes' status was relatively fixed. She did not use the transitory verb form *estar* (to be), which would suggest that indigentes are people who happen to live on the street at this moment (i.e., "están viviendo en la calle" / they are [currently] living on the street or "están sin techo" / they are [currently] homeless). By saying "son de la calle," she suggested that they were (permanently) from the street. Although Clara identified as a radical leftist and health activist, she characterized indigentes as biological, physical, and moral threats to the presumably more legitimate residents of the community. Her discourse marginalized indigentes by describing them in terms that suggested they were categorically different from other people. Although Clara was responsible for the Negra Hipólita center's founding in the first place, she shared residents' alarm at the "spectacle" of their inappropriate behavior. In describing people as naked, violent, and devoid of shame or propriety, Clara echoed media reports that blamed indigentes for the deterioration of public spaces.

Even a pro-poor activist like Clara—who proudly identified herself as belonging to the historically marginalized majority and struggling to build her own home, whose breeze block walls and dirt floors suggested a level of poverty not yet transcended—portrayed indigentes as a class apart from herself and her neighbors. Characterized as possessing different kinds of bodies and morality, indigentes represented threats to the legitimate members of the community. Clara's narrative rationalized the decision to bus them to distant rehabilitation centers. Clara stated categorically, "Here there are no [Negra Hipólita centers], no. They have to be in an outlying area [*retirado de los sectores*], they can't exist inside of a neighborhood [lit., "sector"]."

Caraqueños commonly associated the bodies of indigentes—bodies that were identifiable by their unkempt demeanor, shabby clothes, and behaviors attributable to drug and alcohol abuse—with certain spaces. This happened in two ways. First, residents associated indigentes with the improper use of local spaces (plazas, boulevards, abandoned buildings, parks). Second, residents familiar with government rehabilitation efforts associated the bodies of indigentes with distant bucolic institutions geared specifically to their care. Unlike the public spaces of their own neighborhood, distant institutional settings were seen as the proper spaces for housing and healing indigentes. Even when indigentes participated in the Negra Hipólita program they were likely to elicit displeasure if they stayed in the local community.

When I continued fieldwork in Santa Teresa in 2008 I observed a near-total lack of community activism focused on rehabilitating indigentes. Many of the people who trained with the Negra Hipólita mission in 2006 now worked as community health workers in Barrio Adentro and had stopped doing homeless outreach. When I asked for an update on Negra Hipólita they directed me to a nearby park (Parque Los Caobos) that had a facility to receive people who agreed to get help.

The program continued to operate around the city, evidenced by large painted buses that state employees used for mobile outreach. I visited the site in Los Caobos Park and observed as individuals completed a comprehensive intake process that marked their departure from the streets and entry into the institutional world of the Negra Hipólita mission. New participants stayed at the facility until they were bused to a relatively distant rehabilitation center for long-term treatment. Visibly disheveled people, mostly men, sat in plastic chairs outside a large temporary building while workers gave each one an intake interview, a haircut, and a hot meal in a Styrofoam container. One man received first aid treatment for a head injury and sat eating his food with a white bandage wrapped around his head. Some men who completed intake stood talking to each other around a set of body building bars in the park adjacent to the facility. Hurricane fencing separated the building and a patio area from the rest of the park, where couples strolled and children chased each other around large trees and decorative fountains.

In Santa Teresa the program functioned without the community involvement originally intended. Now specialist teams employed by the government approached potential participants. From here, participants went to the park, then to long-term rehabilitation centers.[14] Somewhat ironically named Centers of Social Inclusion, they were commonly located in rural parts of the country. The national news agency (Agencia Venezolana de Noticias, or AVN) explained:

> Those Venezuelans who choose to change their living situation receive free treatment for ten months with trained personnel to help them discover their potential and develop their talent, a method through which at least four thousand people across the country have accomplished family, labor, and educational reintegration, recovering their human dignity.

Note that official government discourse framed rehabilitation as requiring individual will (Venezuelans must "choose to change their living situation") as well as government aid.

Community members sympathetic to the program mentioned its optimistic aims of social reintegration and dignity less frequently as time passed. One day in one of Santa Teresa's Barrio Adentro clinics, I mentioned to Alejandra and Carlos, the nurse and dentist, that I was planning to visit Los Caobos's Negra Hipólita center. I was surprised when our lighthearted conversation turned serious at my mention of the Negra Hipólita site. Alejandra and Carlos began lecturing me about how I should not go there alone or even with Lilian (who had promised to take me there). Negra Hipólita was very dangerous, they said. The people there were *chiflados* and *asesinos,* crazies and murderers, they exclaimed. If I go I should try to take a big group with me for safety in numbers.

I grew accustomed to Venezuelans warning me away from certain areas of the city because of concerns about violent crime, but it struck me that Alejandra and Carlos would speak this way. People identifiable as *indigentes* frequently came to their clinic as patients. For many months I observed them providing medical services, treating patients with respect and good humor. Each spoke earnestly in other contexts about their commitment to humanitarianism and social justice. Alejandra and Carlos began working for Barrio Adentro when they could have obtained better paid positions elsewhere, because they believed in the cause. Recall Alejandra's claim about caring for all types of patients (chap. 3): "Here there are no class distinctions. Here in Barrio Adentro a patient may come in who's able to pay for a private clinic, all the way down to an indigent who doesn't even have the money to pay for his own bandages in a hospital." So it seemed incongruous that the idea of indigentes evoked fear and displeasure among even humanitarian-minded health workers.

Alejandra and Carlos appeared to hold contradictory views: in their professional roles they viewed indigentes as patients like any other, with equal rights to medical care and dignified treatment, but when advising a foreigner about navigating the city, a view of indigentes as chiflados and asesinos predominated. Alejandra's and Carlos's inconsistency reflected a tension that I sensed among local health activists: they vacillated between a discourse of human rights, social justice, and caring for socially excluded people and a tendency to see indigentes as a different class of people who threatened community well-being.

THE IMPERATIVE TO DEMARGINALIZE

Training in the Negra Hipólita program served as a source of pleasure for people, but the same people expressed discontent, frustration, and sometimes disgust with *los indigentes* once it became clear that the program was not working as imagined. To make sense of this dynamic we must understand the concept of *marginalidad* (marginality; social exclusion) in Bolivarian Venezuela. At the end of the twentieth century increasing numbers of Venezuelans experienced poverty and other forms of social exclusion as the national economy fell into crisis. Chávez won overwhelming popular support by giving voice to the frustration and injustice of social inequality. The foundational narrative of the Chávez government promised that the marginalized majority would gain the opportunity to demarginalize and empower themselves. State officials promised that social inclusion, popular participation, and popular power would result from participating in programs like Negra Hipólita and Barrio Adentro.[15] Nongovernmental organizations like the Pan American Health Organization (the regional body of the World Health Organization) supported this narrative, claiming that government programs like Barrio Adentro would empower the country's poor.[16] I observed neighborhood residents who supported the Chávez government engage in this discourse constantly.

According to this discourse, demarginalization depended on people actively participating in their own transformation. In spite of sweeping government promises to redress social inequalities, much of the responsibility for achieving social inclusion was imagined to rest with marginalized individuals. This is why state media emphasized *la participación del pueblo,* or the participation of the people, in narratives promising social change. The success of social programs depended on whether and to what extent people engaged with them. This helps explain why community members involved in government health projects emphasized the need for mass participación, urging neighbors, acquaintances, and even strangers to participate in a health fair, an exercise class, or a community meeting.

The ideology of demarginalization that undergirded Chávez-era health programs required agentive change at the individual, social, and state level. At the individual level indigentes and activists were expected to transform in ways that made them better citizens.[17] For indigentes this meant making the most of (aprovechando) social services that promised to deliver tangible benefits and exerting individual will to abstain from alcohol and drugs. For activists this meant participating in programs to improve the lives of marginalized others. Demarginalization at the social level involved reintegrating marginalized persons into community affairs, the formal economy, and politics. It entailed recuperating dilapidated spaces such as streets, parks, plazas, and buildings for healthful community use. Both of these processes were expected to unfold when individuals took opportunities to rehabilitate themselves and each other. At the state level demarginalization required government institutions to recognize historically marginalized people as full citizens deserving of care and justice. This form of demarginalization became manifest when government social programs offered tangible benefits to help people reach their full potential.

There was an inherent tension to the value of *marginalización* (marginalization) in Bolivarian Venezuela. People encouraged each other to overcome marginality while simultaneously celebrating a shared identity rooted in a history of marginalization. Members of marginalized groups were framed as properly moral in contrast to elites, who were cast as egotistical, power hungry, and classist. Hence the lack of euphemism in the government naming its health program "Barrio Adentro," even though the word *barrio* has a history of being used in a derogatory manner the way English speakers would use the word *slum* or *shantytown*. In a political moment that valorized the poor and historically marginalized, being from the barrio was something to be proud of, as long as one was making an effort to empower oneself.

Demarginalizing oneself entailed taking advantage of opportunities for social welfare and political inclusion. If you were sick (or even if you felt healthy), you should go to the local Barrio Adentro clinic and get checked out. If you learned about an opportunity to support a local clinic through volunteer work and you had the available free time, you should try to help. You should actively engage in community vitality efforts, such as cleaning up the public plaza or painting a new mural. The logic behind this way of enacting citizenship was presented as commonsensical and taken-for-granted: Why *wouldn't* you want to improve your own health, empower yourself, and create a more livable neighborhood?

Yet, in spite of volunteers' and employees' efforts, many indigentes refused or otherwise failed to engage in government-sponsored rehabilitation. Residents seemed to interpret continued homelessness, drug abuse, and alcohol addiction as indicators that indigentes were unwilling or at least unable to participate in their own demarginalization. Even some Negra Hipólita staff blamed indigentes for a presumed lack of personal will and failure to take responsibility. A shelter director who overcame homelessness and drug addiction himself told a journalist, "They prefer to flee their problems and just say for now they don't want to move forward. For them it just seems easier to continue taking drugs and living on the streets than assuming a level of responsibility."[18]

Because of their nonparticipation in projects of demarginalization and because of their apparent refusal to seek out, demand, or claim benefits and services, indigentes represented a grave threat at several levels. They threatened a dominant model of individual and social change that required people to embrace opportunities for empowerment. And because volunteers' own sense of empowerment and belonging depended on their ability to recruit others to empower themselves, the apparent refusal of indigentes to participate reflected poorly on them.

Political will and government resources could only go so far when models of health and citizenship demanded agentive participation. Expecting people to embrace opportunities to improve their health exhilarated and motivated research participants because it meant they got to actively construct their own state of well-being, their own political belonging, and their own empowerment. But subscribing to this expectation meant that certain groups evoked displeasure for failing to live up to an idealized process of demarginalization.

People's inability to be incorporated successfully into social programs like Misión Negra Hipólita and their continued visibility in public spaces made them everyday reminders that for some the radical promises of the Chávez government to eradicate inequality were not being met. The nonparticipation of indigentes highlighted the inevitable incompleteness of revolutionary projects. Because the ideological stakes of participation were so high, indigentes who failed to engage in practices of self-transformation were seen to flaunt moral imperatives of citizenship.

The anthropologist Mary Douglas's classic analysis in her book *Purity and Danger* helps explain why indigentes evoked displeasure among activists who initially sympathized with their suffering. Douglas explained that "persons in a marginal state . . . who are somehow left out of the patterning of society" pose a threat to social order.[19] Classic examples of marginal persons are prisoners and psychiatric patients, whose marginality is manifested in their abnormal behavior and their residence in institutional settings.[20] People in the margins represent a danger to the overall orderliness of a social system. Incorporating them is difficult, sometimes impossible.

In Bolivarian Venezuela simply belonging to a marginal group did not threaten the social order. During the Chávez era the dominant historical narrative of the Venezuelan nation-state normalized social marginality. Marginality was a product of structural forces that could be reversed. It became acceptable to be marginal; in fact, it became something to be proud of. However, what did threaten the social order was not trying to fix one's own marginality. Because indigentes rejected available sources of care and personal transformation, they appeared complicit in their own continued marginality, undercutting the political discourse of demarginalization and empowerment. The problem was not marginality itself, as Douglas posited, but rather a marginality that resisted recuperation. For residents celebrating positive social change through demarginalization, the body of the indigente represented physical and political danger. In addition to threatening the harmony and cleanliness of public spaces, persistent street homelessness endangered idealized notions of demarginalization and citizenship. This is a central reason why volunteers' sympathy gave way to frustration and anger as they learned how difficult it could be to help indigentes. When rehabilitation efforts did not follow idealized scripts, residents directed displeasure and even disgust at the bodies of indigentes. Volunteers' displeasure with indigentes expressed political dissatisfaction over incomplete processes of demarginalization.

The philosopher Slavoj Žižek's theory of national identity as a form of enjoyment helps explain why Venezuelan activists found indigentes so displeasing. Žižek argues that national identity is important to people because it serves as a source of pleasure. Nations are meaningful not because they consolidate a supposedly essential ethnic identity but rather because they help people "organize their enjoyment."[21] National identity is about "the way subjects of a given ethnic community organize their enjoyment through national myths." Žižek argues that racism and xenophobic nationalism permeate democratic nation-states because ethnic "others" threaten the pleasure offered by myths of national belonging. As he puts it, "We always impute to the 'other' an excessive enjoyment: he wants to steal our enjoyment (by ruining our way of life)."[22] Caracas's indigentes were not an ethnic "other," but they certainly appeared as others compared to everyone else. Applying Žižek's argument to this case, we could say that indigentes' refusal to demarginalize themselves according to idealized scripts represented a "theft of enjoyment" because it threatened a national myth of health and empowerment. Even at the mundane level of everyday life, street homelessness viscerally threatened the pleasure people sought from community public spaces.

In the case of Negra Hipólita, a potentially uplifting model of healing contained within its own utopian vision limits on national belonging. Domestic politics under Chávez focused on reversing social, political, and economic marginality. Poor and working-class Venezuelans celebrated opportunities for participation in empowering health programs. But not everybody was able or willing to participate in idealized ways. Indigentes evoked displeasure by exposing the limits of a model of citizenship that required people to demarginalize themselves.

The case of Negra Hipólita shows how imperatives to demarginalize oneself and embrace a new citizenship status can have unintended consequences. Deeply marginalized people presented with opportunities to improve their health and their position in the social order who did not take up these opportunities as expected actually rendered themselves vulnerable to further marginalization. Those who refused rehabilitation services were left to their own devices, openly criticized, and rendered vulnerable to forced removal from spaces they used as shelter, often by the people who volunteered to help them. This turn of events was motivated by the moral threat posed by failing to engage with popular imperatives of empowerment.

This case demonstrates just how important agentive participation was to emergent models of government-provided health care in Bolivarian Venezuela. In a society that attached aesthetic and political significance to seeking out health care, people who failed to engage in health care also failed to behave as proper citizens.

Conclusion

I WROTE THIS BOOK ABOUT THE PLEASURES of government medicine after noticing how this finding consistently surprised people outside of Venezuela, even other medical anthropologists. "Why are they so happy, Amy?," a graduate adviser used to ask me, over and over. What was obvious to research participants and manifestly observable by me as an ethnographer was not obvious to people outside Bolivarian Venezuela. Poor and working-class Caraqueños took pleasure in government health programs because these programs disrupted existing power dynamics. They empowered people—literally empowered their bodies—by improving their sense of biophysical health. Just as important, Barrio Adentro empowered people politically by recognizing them as people who mattered. Expressions of pleasure communicated people's subjective understanding that things were changing for the better.

Empowerment was not a zero-sum game where some people won power and others lost out. Instead, research participants felt themselves becoming more physically vital, more respected by the government, more valued in society at large, and more equal vis-à-vis the historically entrenched elite. In this political moment, a sense of empowerment unfolded across multiple domains, not just health care. Government programs allowed people to experience empowerment through local governance, community food schemes, education, and media production. People's excitement about government health care was inseparable from a broader sense of buoyed spirits at seeing a state doing what it had long promised to do: redistribute the profits of Venezuela's oil to Venezuela's people.

In Bolivarian Venezuela health care tangibly fulfilled state promises to "sow the oil" and repay the social debt incurred by neoliberalism to improve people's lives. Beyond medical benefits, health services performed political work by recognizing the poor and working classes as part of a social pact that enacted national belonging. Recognition from the state in the form of medical services was important because by marking people as deserving of state resources and care, it marked people as belonging in politically meaningful ways. Venezuelan history established specific conditions under which government health care presented itself as a valued resource and a source of empowerment. Sharing in the country's oil wealth meant enjoying the benefits of citizenship.

In revolutionary Venezuela, government health care effected these changes by responding to cultural desires for compassionate, community-based medicine that complemented existing practices of medical pluralism. Specifically, people took pleasure in the political effects of accessing government health care

- in their neighborhood (chap. 2)
- from an egalitarian and "humanitarian" doctor (chap. 3)
- on their own terms while continuing to practice medical pluralism (chap. 4)
- for others by becoming activists (chaps. 5, 6)
- as participants in health promotion with others in public space (chap. 5)

Empowerment via government medicine depended on people engaging with health programs in particular ways. Health programs called for conscious participation, whether agentively seeking out particular clinics or doctors, maintaining complex routines of medical practices, or developing a new identity as a community activist. The concept of participación itself acquired new meaning as government officials promised a radical reordering of society if people took part in their programs. Research participants generally viewed the moral imperative to participate as a good thing because it put the power to change society in their hands. The notion of building a more participatory democracy appealed to people who felt sidelined by formal politics. But the flip side of this logic was that people who failed to participate as expected could threaten the revolutionary project of social justice and subject themselves to further marginalization.

Many aspects of health care that elicited pleasure among research participants would fail to resonate in a different context, raising questions about how the book's argument applies to other settings. The first time I presented findings from this research in the United States, a famous anthropologist raised her hand and expressed puzzlement that poor Venezuelans might desire intimacy in medical encounters. "I don't want my doctor to give me a hug," she declared, causing the audience to titter. The anthropologist's bemusement at people wanting compassionate touch from a government doctor underlined how class and culture shapes desires for certain forms of health care. The anthropologist, a tenured U.S. academic at a globally renowned university, shared neither class position nor cultural background with Venezuelan research participants, who insisted that doctors express love and solidarity. We can assume that for the anthropologist, stable employment and finances made access to biomedicine a taken-for-granted part of life. She would have health insurance through work and not have to look to the government for access to health care. The anthropologist's privileged class position meant she was unlikely to view doctors as symbols of a caring state or to invest medical encounters with political significance. For her, doctors improved biophysical health but probably did not index the kind of political inclusion that this book has analyzed.

In the United States, the dominant cultural model of a good doctor prioritizes technical competence over caring qualities so much that an uncaring misanthrope might still be considered a good doctor given sufficient technical expertise.[1] Venezuelan research participants would find this absurd.[2] Also, U.S. ideologies of bootstrapping and rugged individualism inform a model of state-citizen relations in which accessing government social services represents a failure of personal responsibility, and people who use such services are stigmatized as state "dependents."[3] In contrast, Venezuelans understand citizenship as sharing national oil wealth through government projects, meaning that state-distributed resources appear as a birthright rather than as a mark of shame.

In commenting on the uniqueness of people's desires for compassionate touch in a biomedical setting, the anthropologist drew attention to the contingent aspects of the Venezuelan case. Pleasure produced by a doctor expressing love for her patients was a contingent experience, possible only because cultural and historical circumstances made these actions desirable in the first place. This book shows that empowerment through health care depended on specific medical policies and practices aligning with local desires.

However, for as much as it seems culturally and historically unique, this book helps explain responses to health care cross-culturally. Barrio Adentro took hold in a democratic nation-state whose people were divided by social inequalities and vulnerable to the forces of global capitalism. As in many other societies, state officials asserted a commitment to the idea of social welfare, establishing expectations that one of the things governments did was provide social benefits to promote equality and improve people's lives. We should not be puzzled to see poor and working-class people in this setting take pleasure in suddenly receiving valued resources like health care. When a government follows through on promises to redress social inequalities by providing valued forms of social welfare, we should not be puzzled to see poor and working-class people express a level of excitement that reflects more than just happiness about the material benefits.

A DECADE LATER

The years I conducted fieldwork (2006–9) represented a high point in the Chávez government's expansion of social programs. The country enjoyed a booming economy thanks to historically high global oil prices. The political will of the Venezuelan state was literally etched into the urban landscape in the form of Barrio Adentro clinics, octagonal structures with bright blue edges that popped out of the background. Even then, some people expressed concern about the durability of my research findings, based on the assumption that observations made during a period of revolutionary change were too ephemeral to provide lasting insights. Since that period much has changed. The government of Chávez's successor, Nicolás Maduro, continued to endorse revolution via projects like Barrio Adentro but struggled to provide material benefits. Today political and economic uncertainties threaten to overwhelm Venezuelan society, raising questions about the long-term relevance of this book's argument. Some people have asked whether I can predict a fundamentally unpredictable future (e.g., "What happens to Barrio Adentro if a right-wing candidate becomes president?"). Others have suggested that the unpredictability of Venezuelan politics and economy negates any claims I am making. Drawing on narratives of instability common in analyses of Latin America, people have questioned the durability of research findings by citing the doomed nature of single-export economies, socialism, populism, or authoritarian leadership. Regardless of whether we agree with such critiques, these comments underline the fact that Venezuelan people have experienced economic and political life as unstable for decades. Societies constantly undergo change—no society exists frozen in time—but in Venezuela rapid social change and ongoing instability has made the future appear particularly uncertain.

Ten years have passed since the beginning of long-term fieldwork on this project, and much has changed. I write this conclusion in early 2018, dismayed by the increasingly unstable conditions of life in Venezuela. Since Chávez's death in 2013, the government of his elected successor, Maduro, has failed to heal social divisions or ease economic woes brought on by a fall in the global price of oil. A violent right-wing opposition demands regime change but offers few ideas for how to govern. Global media coverage of Venezuela paints a grim picture of economic crisis, political protests, government repression, and authoritarianism and debates the need for foreign intervention. In spite of giving the crisis significant media attention, journalists rarely explain why the opposition has failed to win support among those hit hardest. The following discussion offers a view of the contemporary moment from the perspective of poor and working-class Venezuelans, based on recent conversations with research participants and analyses by anthropologists, sociologists, and historians of Venezuela.[4]

Venezuelans suffered a significant decline in living conditions starting around 2014. The vagaries of global capitalism, economic mismanagement, corruption, speculation, and corporate hoarding all played a role. On top of this, the country's historical dependence on oil exports made it practically impossible to avoid economic crisis at this moment. With an economy tied to a wildly fluctuating market for oil, the Venezuelan government has been vulnerable to boom and bust cycles. Oil dependency predates the leftist leadership of Maduro and Chávez, but Maduro's government acted in ways that worsened the effects of the economic downturn. Failing to reform currency controls contributed to inflation rates as high as 800 percent, making daily activities like ATM withdrawals and grocery shopping exercises in absurdity. Also a legacy of oil dependence, the country contends with a historical dependence on imported rather than domestically produced food. This becomes particularly problematic during periods of high inflation, when purchasing power shrinks. Many companies and private individuals took advantage of currency regulations and price controls (meant to make food and basic goods affordable) to engage in hoarding and speculation on a massive scale, contributing to scarcity and a costly black market for necessities. Inflation and shortages of food, basic goods, and medications affected everybody, especially those with limited incomes who lacked access to U.S. dollars.

People often spent hours a day obtaining necessities, and many lost weight due to food insecurity. In 2017 a friend who works for a government agency in Caracas told me things were so bad she saw people eating out of trash cans on a daily basis.

Venezuelans also are suffering a political crisis that affects everyday life viscerally. In addition to ineffectual and corrupt governance under Maduro (charges made by many on the Left and the Right), his administration recently made decisions that undermined nearly twenty years of participatory democracy, including suspending regional elections, suspending a recall referendum process, and (briefly) dissolving the National Assembly. The right-wing opposition denounced Maduro's government for being antidemocratic and repressive. Yet their own actions belied a commitment to democracy and rule of law. Opposition leaders called for replacing the democratically elected government by any means necessary, and opposition protests (some intentionally violent) wreaked havoc in Caracas. Some protesters built burning barricades to impede traffic, strung wire across roads to cause bodily harm (at least one motorcyclist was beheaded in this way), attacked government food centers and medical clinics, and, in at least three instances, burned people alive for looking "chavista" (i.e., poor and brown-skinned). Over one hundred people died in incidents related to protests and looting over a five-month period in 2017. Police forces, opposition protesters, and pro-government actors have all been implicated in these deaths.[5] Attempts at dialogue between government and opposition leaders have failed, leaving little hope for a compromise to ease the crisis.

In early 2018, frustration and exhaustion (*desgaste,* a wearing down over time) hung over the city like a fog. The buoyant optimism that animated activists and ordinary people to support government social programs a decade ago has given way to disillusionment. In failing to address an ongoing economic crisis and shoring up their own power at the expense of the people's well-being, government officials have largely abandoned the people they claim to represent. Many continue to support Maduro even though they have lost faith in his government, because the political alternative appeals even less. Historically, right-wing opposition to Chávez and Maduro reflected the interests of the privileged while displaying indifference or even hostility toward poor and racially marginalized Venezuelans. Many Caraqueños are suspicious of a right-wing opposition offering no clear plan for governance whose primary grievances (i.e., state repression, lack of political representation) do not resonate with their own concerns. This was a core reason why opposition protests remained circumscribed in middle- and upper-class neighborhoods. In spite of their frustrations and arguably deeper suffering, historically marginalized residents of the city have not joined protests calling for the government to step down. But barrio residents were not shy about expressing their discontent, denouncing misgovernment through neighborhood protests and cases of looting. One research participant summarized the political situation in Caracas: "Both the government and the opposition are out of touch with our reality."[6]

Amid the crisis, poor and working-class Caraqueños live their lives as well as possible. What choice do they have? The Grandparents Club I attended during fieldwork continued to meet for dance therapy classes and field trips, which they document on Facebook. Last year, as Christmas approached, they organized a holiday party with traditional savory treats like *hallacas,* though the ingredients were much harder to obtain. Many activists and community organizers who received state support and felt empowered during the Chávez era continued to collaborate at the local level through Chávez-era governance structures like communal councils. Even more people continued to identify with Chávez and his visions for radical social change. But many have stopped participating in activist efforts, like Magdalena, who reported that she got discouraged in the years after Chávez died and now focuses her energy on her family rather than community health work.

Given an economic and political crisis affecting all aspects of life, we should not be surprised to learn that people's health has declined since 2008. Especially when compared to just a few years ago, Venezuelans' health and medical services are in grim condition.[7] Food insecurity has affected most Venezuelans, with adverse effects on bodily health and subjective assessments of well-being. A national survey found that 32 percent of respondents ate two or fewer meals per day in 2016 (this is a huge increase from 2015, when 11 percent said they ate two or fewer meals per day).[8] Three of four respondents said they lost weight over the past year. Children were suffering from malnutrition at much higher rates than before, and imported basics like baby formula were scarce and very expensive. People found it very hard to access health care due to shortages of medications, supplies, and equipment, which were largely imported. Medical workers struggled to care for patients amid the scarcity, made worse by ongoing corruption among some hospital workers. In 2017 the health minister was fired after she released data on rising rates of maternal and infant mortality, diphtheria, and malaria. A trusted friend in Caracas explained:

Vaccines for children and adults are scarce or nonexistent, and outbreaks of illnesses like diphtheria are really happening. The situation with respect to health is terrible: you cannot get medications, private health centers have closed down and public ones don't have the supplies to attend to patients. Not even the CDIs [Barrio Adentro diagnostic centers] have medication for high blood pressure, diabetes, etc. The antibiotics that make it into the country, when you can find them, cost almost a month's salary. In reality we are in crisis. Everything has gotten so much worse just in the past few years.

Violent members of the right-wing opposition have made accessing health care not just difficult but also dangerous, attacking government hospitals and Barrio Adentro neighborhood clinics to render them inoperable. Domestic terrorism against government health centers included an opposition-organized siege of a maternity hospital in Miranda state in which burning barricades prevented staff from entering or leaving, forcing a woman in labor and newborns to be evacuated due to risk of smoke inhalation.[9] In Caracas more than fifty children were evacuated from a maternity and children's hospital after armed opposition groups threw stones, started a fire, and stormed the hospital entrance.[10] Barrio Adentro clinics have been ransacked and subjected to attempted arson by opposition protesters.

People explained to me that Barrio Adentro clinics remained open, providing consultations and medications when they were in stock. Katerina said she went to the nearby Barrio Adentro clinic in Santa Teresa twice in 2017, once for medication to treat a migraine (which they did not have) and once with her sister who was sick and needed antibiotics (which they did have). In describing the former experience, she commented on the nurse's disposition even though she did not receive any treatment: "I had to go and buy the migraine medication, but nevertheless the nurse was *amable* [nice, friendly]." Another informant named Yanireth told me she visited her local Barrio Adentro clinic in October 2017 for "a high blood pressure emergency"; she said, "The attention they provided was very good, and they gave me the medication for [hyper]tension." Others also reported that medications and supplies were now scarce. Katerina described Barrio Adentro as "halfway functioning" because medications only arrived sporadically. Magdalena agreed. They said that the number of clinics has increased over the past decade and the demographics of medical workers has shifted as Venezuelans completing medical training through the program began to replace Cuban doctors. These firsthand patient reports suggest that Barrio Adentro remained a government priority in spite of the ongoing crisis.[11]

Although Barrio Adentro operates under severe constraints, it may still serve as a source of pleasure for participants. In describing an encounter with Barrio Adentro in 2017, Magdalena commented on the quality of medical care on display. She wrote:

> This year I visited a CDI and a Barrio Adentro neighborhood clinic. I had a virus that caused an old allergic syndrome to return, which bothered me for two months (note: in the CDI the majority of the doctors are Cuban, with Venezuelan nurses who work with a ton of dedication). I visited the Barrio Adentro neighborhood clinic on September 1, 2017, so they could review the X-ray I got at the CDI in August. They gave me a diagnosis, which was that I had an allergy due to spores, smoke, very strong odors, and other things. The care provided by the doctor was excellent.

Magdalena referred to this visit when I asked for an update on the government's program of medical training for Barrio Adentro.

> With respect to my opinion on [Barrio Adentro] medical training, I will comment on what I saw and heard the day I had my X-ray reviewed. The Cuban doctor who took care of me was with two students in his office. He started by asking me what happened. Then he took the X-ray and started to teach. I was fascinated. He talked to me about my symptoms and why I was coughing so much and how it was making me tired and fatigued. He talked to the medical students about the syndrome and how it manifested. And [he taught them] the hands-on bodily contact required for a doctor to confirm the diagnosis.

I think Magdalena volunteered these details because she knew the dominant media narrative abroad depicted a nonfunctioning health system, which from her perspective was a distortion of reality. Her presentation of this event also suggests that she took pleasure in the encounter. Perhaps she enjoyed Barrio Adentro's style of medical care in 2017 for somewhat different reasons than before. I wonder if she took pleasure in the program in this time of political and economic crisis simply because, against the odds, it continued to exist, showing that the government was at least partially fulfilling former commitments to health. Even when medications were scarce, medical workers could still acknowledge people's dignity and deservingness in clinical consultation.

However, the truth is that in 2017 nobody enjoyed abundant free medical care like what I documented in 2008 and 2009, and caring interactions with doctors cannot make up for the fact that people lack access to lifesaving medicines and their children risk infection because vaccines are in short supply. When access to health care shapes one's quality of life (and life itself, in many cases), it matters little whether the government cannot ensure access due to forces outside its control or because of its own ineptitude. And when health care symbolizes government-sponsored inclusion and empowerment for marginalized people, a lack of health care suggests a rupture in the process of building a more just society.

LOOKING OUTWARD, LOOKING FORWARD

The situation in Venezuela is changing rapidly. By the time you read this, people's living conditions are bound to have changed even more. The analyses presented in this book were based on observations in a political and economic context that no longer exists. The experiences of medically derived pleasure and empowerment that I documented were contingent, but perhaps such is true of all such experiences. An ethnography of Caracas today would produce different descriptions of people's experiences of health care, but it would not invalidate what I observed or concluded. Ethnography asks us to understand people's lives in the context of messy historical contingencies, in order to make claims about humanity that resonate beyond that specific culture or era. The inevitability of historical change does not invalidate arguments about human experience grounded in particular sociocultural and historical contexts. This book argues that particular forms of government medicine can produce pleasure and empowerment by making people feel recognized, cared for, and valued. If something significant changes about that government or its health care, we should anticipate different outcomes.

I hope these research findings invite speculation and spark discussions beyond the central themes of the book. In the final pages I consider how this book could be read for insights on health policy and the study of political revolutions. Looking forward, I also comment on what the ethnography suggests about the long-term legacy of Chávez-era social programs.

Health Policy

For people involved in health policy work, this book underlines the need to institute and evaluate medical interventions in cultural context. Some insights reinforce recommendations that medical anthropologists have been making for years but often go unheeded by policy makers. For example, one-size-fits-all solutions to health care make little sense when public reception depends so heavily on local expectations shaped by historical specificities. Clinical care represents a microcosm of social relations writ large, with power to reinforce or destabilize how patients perceive their position in the social order. Perceptions of deservingness shape demands for, and reactions to, different kinds of medical care.

The Venezuelan case also reveals that viewing affective responses to health care as noise that gets in the way of determining a program's real effects on health is misguided. Expressions of pleasure and displeasure provide insights into the meanings people attach to experiences of medicine. These meanings shape people's likelihood of using medical care (rather than avoiding it), celebrating a health intervention (rather than denigrating it), and assessing their own health as improving (rather than worsening).

Health policies should complement biophysical measures of health with a contextualized view of medicine that takes participants' realities seriously. This requires a less paternalistic approach to health policy in favor of approaches that acknowledge the sensibility and validity of people's desires regarding health care. If we were to apply the book's findings to predict the effectiveness of a prospective health policy, we could ask, Where is care provided, and how is the physical location of services meaningful for patients? Who provides care, what kind of relationship do they cultivate with patients, and why does this matter? How do medical authorities in this milieu relate to nondominant healing traditions, and how will this influence patient engagement with the prospective policy? To what extent are patients drawn into the health policy as agents of change versus treated as recipients of services in a top-down fashion, and how does this align with local desires? To what extent does the policy promise to enact social transformations beyond providing medical care, and do such promises resonate with local concerns?

Political Revolution

Societies undergoing political revolution provide an opportunity to learn how people imagine, create, and experience radical sociopolitical change, yet anthropologists have published few ethnographic accounts of revolution.[12] By "revolution," I mean a rapid reworking of a society's core political and ideological formations, impelled by mass popular support and by leaders who destabilize existing power structures.[13] We have few ethnographies of revolution, partly for pragmatic reasons. Political revolutions may entail widespread violence; most anthropologists do not want to risk their lives collecting data. Agencies that fund anthropologists often refuse to fund research in countries they deem politically unstable. Ethnographic projects may require years of preparatory work (language training, grant applications, developing contacts, etc.) before fieldwork begins, while revolutionary moments can arise without warning and dissipate just as quickly.

Logistical challenges aside, certain biases deter anthropologists from studying revolution. Early generations of professional anthropologists studied small-scale, non-Western societies, producing ethnographies that portrayed people and cultures as "frozen in time" even when societies were undergoing tumultuous change due to colonization. Anthropologists now take for granted that no society is static, yet the idea that ethnographies should examine relatively stable settings continues to influence our choice of field sites and the advice graduate students receive. Trying to analyze a society undergoing rapid change is daunting because what we observe could change at any moment.[14]

In addition, our skepticism about the potential for profound social transformation (such as an end to capitalism) limits our ability to take revolutionary movements seriously as objects of study. As the anthropologist Alpa Shah said in her 2012 Malinowski Memorial Lecture, "Our lack of attention to attempts at shaping radically different visions of the future in the present is perhaps a reflection of a more general disillusionment with concepts of utopia as being untenable."[15] While anthropologists strongly sympathize with struggles for social justice that manifest as protest and resistance "from below," we have become quite jaded when it comes to state-led social transformations, grand narratives of progress, and utopian visions of the future.

Conducting research under these circumstances requires changing our mind-set about what ethnography can and should achieve. Anthropology shows how humans have created radically different forms of life—different economic systems, interactions with our environment, social relations, and spiritual worlds. We are theoretically and methodologically well situated to examine how people re-create radically different forms of life. Ethnographic research on revolutions could address how people come to believe in a different future, what conditions are needed to activate (and sustain) a popular imaginary committed to comprehensive social transformation, and what kinds of popular mobilizations produce lasting change. Examining actual attempts to forge deep social and political transformation would help us better understand what it takes to enact broad-scale, popularly supported structural change.

We can read this book as an anthropological study of revolution. The analysis contributes an ethnographic understanding of life in times of revolution by showing the importance of positive experiences of pleasure, joy, and satisfaction. Positive affective experiences of government programs sustained people's belief that another world was possible and motivated many to collaborate in building a radically different future. These findings suggest that pleasure and fun serve as important guiding ethics for political revolution. We should examine positive affective experiences associated with times of radical political change, as they may play a major role in mobilizing popular involvement. Observing playful engagement in political rallies and activist work in Caracas, I wondered to what degree pleasure motivates participation in revolution. I also wondered whether it was a coincidence that in this setting self-sacrifice as a guiding ethos for building socialism was practically nonexistent. In contrast to other revolutionary societies (like Cuba), the suggestion that poor and working-class Venezuelans needed to sacrifice their material needs and wants for the greater good or for a better future was not at all salient. These observations point to some directions that future anthropological research on revolution might take.

Barrio Adentro's Legacy

For decades Latin Americans protested neoliberalism and imagined postneoliberal futures promising greater social equality. Much of Latin America experienced democratically elected Left leadership during the first decade of the 2000s, with Venezuela one of the more long-lasting and uplifting examples of leftist government. Even as chaotic economic and political problems put the country's future in question, we should speculate about which developments arising from the Chávez era, specifically from Barrio Adentro, are likely to endure.

My observations (and those of other researchers) suggest that as a result of the Bolivarian Revolution, the majority of Venezuelans have become accustomed to state-citizen relations grounded in reciprocity and the promise of sociopolitical empowerment. By reciprocity, I mean modes of government and citizenship in which a state provides (or aims to provide) for people's wants and needs and people reciprocate by playing a substantive role in governance. Both sides of this reciprocal relationship can produce a sense of empowerment, which in turn can magnify people's sense of entitlement to this pattern of state-citizen relations. While these expectations and desires predated Chávez and created the conditions for Chávez's rise to power, under his leadership the state manifested as a reciprocal, empowering form of government different from the ones that came before.

Zoraida, a middle-class administrator for a social services organization, explained how the revolutionary government changed people's understandings of political power and their relationship with the state.

> I remember in the seventies and eighties, we were an apathetic people, indifferent to everything. We didn't know about and didn't care about voting, nothing was important to us. If someone gave us a kilo of rice for a vote, that was all well and good, but nobody really cared about anything, you know? In contrast, this government has helped produce an awakening for people, telling us, "Look, those of you who have an indigenous background also have rights, and the grandparents have rights, and women have rights, and street children have rights." We're not quite there yet, but we're getting there, you know?

Zoraida distinguished between simply receiving government benefits and feeling entitled to, empowered by, and deserving of government benefits. She refers to being uplifted and "awakened" by a government that recognizes the deservingness of historically marginalized Venezuelans.

Barrio Adentro instantiated a state-citizen dynamic defined by reciprocity and empowerment. I predict poor and working-class Venezuelans will feel entitled to this form of government even in the face of continued economic hardship or a dramatic change of leadership. After fifteen years of Barrio Adentro, people believe that they have the right to empathic and community-based medicine and that they have the right to play an active role in improving health in their neighborhoods. These expectations will drive demands and desires for politically empowering government medicine well into the future. Gabriella, one of Santa Teresa's middle-aged community health workers and a student of community development at the government's Bolivarian University of Venezuela, said this more eloquently than I could. I end by sharing her speculations on her country's future.

> This political vision of the president's might be lost, because we might not have this president in the future. We might lose *chavismo,* but the vision of an empowered *pueblo,* this will not be lost. . . . It is we who are going to make demands, it is we who will really struggle. We are going to achieve what we really want. We'll always have difficulties, but we'll be working towards what we want. When you write your book, say that it will be this way.

NOTES

CHAPTER ONE

1. In Venezuela, barrios, often translated into English as "slums," are poor neighborhoods made up of irregular landholdings and informal housing, historically located in urban peripheries and lacking key government services.

2. All names are pseudonyms.

3. In the book I provide currency conversions based on the 2008 official exchange rate of 2.15 Venezuelan bolivares (Bs) to 1 U.S. dollar (US$). However, the unofficial exchange rate was approximately 5 Bs to US$1. Speakers who refer to millions of bolivares were using predevaluation terminology. On January 1, 2008, the bolívar was officially devalued/replaced at rate of 1 to 1,000.

4. My use of the term "biomedicine" implies a cohesive medical system, though biomedicine takes heterogeneous forms that vary even within the same society (e.g., the distinct biomedical traditions in Venezuela before and after Barrio Adentro).

5. For example, the anthropologist Vania Smith-Oka found that low-income indigenous women giving birth in a public hospital in Mexico experienced agonizing and medically unnecessary cervical exams as well as verbal threats to control their cries of pain. She notes that this callous and coercive treatment reflected "a pattern of disdain and humiliation [that] exists in many public hospitals across Mexico. . . . [T]he patients in my study knew that this hospital was 'a place for the poor' and that they would not get the sort of treatment they would at a private institution" (Smith-Oka 2013, 601; see also Smith-Oka 2012; Vega 2018). Ethnographic accounts reporting similar findings for other countries include Nicole Berry's research in Guatemala (Berry 2012, 2008), Catherine Maternowska's research in Haiti (Maternowska 2006), Nancy Scheper-Hughes's work in Brazil (1993), and Marilyn Nations's and Linda-Anne Rebhun's work in Brazil (1988).

6. For example, McCallum and dos Reis argue that in the public hospital where they conducted fieldwork in Salvador, Brazil, births "powerfully construct race and class differences, ordered through the asymmetrical social relationships that govern the hospital birth process. In its day-to-day dramas, the hospital distils the social

differences between poor, black women and white, middle-class professionals into a highly concentrated form … [that] sustain[s] the social order both within and outside of the institution's walls" (2005, 355).

7. Briggs and Mantini-Briggs 2003, 10. See also their more recent work, Briggs and Mantini-Briggs 2016.

8. Briggs and Mantini-Briggs 2003, 10–11.

9. Martinez 2005, 806.

10. Many ethnographies of public health care in Latin America document treatment that people would want to avoid. Alexander Edmonds describes Brazilian public hospitals as "poorly funded and often beset by long lines, crumbling infrastructure, and rude service" (Edmonds 2012, 4). Dominique Béhague and colleagues found that poor and middle-class Brazilian research participants tried hard to avoid the low-quality care and neglect associated with public hospital births (Béhague 2002; Béhague, Victoria, and Barros 2002). Elizabeth Roberts's work among Ecuadorian IVF patients revealed that "even poor and working-class families spent large amounts of their own resources in order to avoid public services" (Roberts 2012, 23). Trying to understand why Haitians avoided a well-funded and accessible family planning clinic despite their stated desires to have fewer children, Catherine Maternowska documented clinical practices in which "clients are objectified and treatment depersonalized, devoid of respect or dignity. … It was not uncommon to see nurses and doctors physically recoil when more destitute clients were in need of services. It was as if they were repulsive. … Doctors would typically deliver rapid orders in stern and loud voices, full of disdain, while women timidly and nervously undressed. 'Take off your underwear, take them off. Not your skirt, just get the underwear! Off!' … They often left the clinic with unresolved problems, or worse, misunderstandings regarding their health" (Maternowska 2006, 78–97).

11. Exceptions include Alyssa Bernstein's research on Cuban medical training in Bolivia (Bernstein 2013), Emily Yates-Doerr's work on women's interactions with government nutritionists in Guatemala (Yates-Doerr 2012), and Alex Nading's analysis of Nicaraguan community health workers engaging in mosquito control efforts (Nading 2012). These studies document pleasurable dimensions of government health care, and Nading makes pleasure the focus of analysis.

12. Farquhar 1994, 471.

13. Ortner 2016, 47.

14. Ortner was not the first to document this trend in anthropology. A small but controversial set of commentaries has critiqued what Ortner calls "dark anthropology" (note that Ortner herself does not critique this research, nor do I). Some scholars question the motivations of researchers who study suffering and disempowerment, suggesting, for example, that ethnographies of suffering are a kind of "voyeuristic quasi-pornography" (Kelly 2013, 214) and that studying the powerless allows us to take pleasure in our own self-righteousness (Kulick 2006). Other scholars question the effects of research on suffering. Some claim that studies of "the suffering subject" or "the suffering stranger" undermine anthropological inquiry by stripping away cultural and historical specificities of people's lives to present a

decontextualized universal humanity with which we are invited to empathize (see Robbins 2013; Butt 2002). Referring to recent scholarship on poor urban and Native communities, Eve Tuck critiques what she calls "damage-centered research" that "looks to historical exploitation, domination, and colonization to explain contemporary brokenness, such as poverty, poor health, and low literacy," suggesting that "the danger in damage-centered research is that it is a pathologizing approach in which the oppression singularly defines a community" (Tuck 2009, 413). Some of these critics have called for more research on the positive aspects of social life, especially in marginalized communities, noting that anthropology's interest in disempowerment and inequality may have inadvertently foreclosed studying and writing about "the good" (see Han 2013 for a response to this kind of critique).

15. Race 2009, 2017.

16. Peterson, Nørgaard, and Traulsen 2015; Keane 2008.

17. Trnka 2017; Naraindas and Bastos 2011.

18. Mitchell 2001; Georges 2008; Mitchell and Georges 1997; Harris et al. 2004.

19. Farquhar 1994.

20. Farquhar and Zhang 2005, 2012.

21. Yates-Doerr 2012; Roberts 2012a, 2012b; Nading 2012. Also see Halliburton 2003.

22. Race 2009, 9.

23. Anthropologists have begun to focus more explicitly on happiness, well-being, and pleasure in recent years. See, e.g., the special issue of *Hau: Journal of Ethnographic Theory* titled "Happiness: Horizons of Purpose" (Kavedzija and Walker 2015); the Vital Topics Forum in *American Anthropologist* titled "On Happiness" (Johnston et al. 2012); and the books *Pursuits of Happiness: Well-Being in Anthropological Perspective* (Mathews and Izquierdo 2009) and *The Good Life: Aspiration, Dignity, and the Anthropology of Wellbeing* (Fischer 2014).

24. Coronil 1997.

25. In her ethnography of midwifery among African Americans in the South, Gertrude Fraser notes that "medicalization of childbirth was, on the whole, seen as a positive occurrence," partly because it entailed inclusion in a public health apparatus from which this population had been historically marginalized. She says, "Reproductive change signaled African Americans' symbolic, if not fully realized, inclusion in the field of vision of a health care bureaucracy that had until then largely ignored their health needs. If this meant giving up the much-valued midwife, it could also lead to being a part of the 'public' in public health" (Fraser 1998, 177–78).

26. See Tinker Salas 2009.

27. The anthropologist Fernando Coronil noted that early notions of Venezuelan citizenship never reflected classical liberal ideas of a rights-bearing individual maximizing their interests in a free market. Instead, "the citizen was construed as a member of a corporate national body, not just as the autonomous agent of an atomized market or as the isolated bearer of formal rights.... [D]emocracy [was understood] as the extension of social participation not only in national politics but also in the national wealth" (Coronil 1997, 88).

28. OPS 2006.

29. Ellner and Salas 2005 critically evaluates this theory.

30. Tinker Salas 2015.

31. See Ciccariello-Maher 2013 for a history of Venezuelan social movements and revolutionary groups that predated and laid the foundations for Chávez's emergence as a leftist politician.

32. Hellinger and Melcher 1998.

33. OPS 2006.

34. This study was undertaken by Rakowski and Kastner (1985) for the Institute of Advanced Management Studies in Caracas.

35. Coronil 1997.

36. Harvey 2005; Ganti 2014; Brown 2015.

37. Coronil 1997; Ellner 2008.

38. Lander and Fierro 1996.

39. Rates of extreme poverty rose during this period from 11% to 34% (Lander and Fierro 1996).

40. Armada et al. 2009; Briggs and Mantini-Briggs 2009.

41. Lander and Fierro 1996; OPS 2006. One estimate suggests that infant mortality rates nearly doubled between 1988 and 1990 (Hellinger and Melcher 1998).

42. Villasana López 2010.

43. Lander 2005.

44. Schemo 1998, quoted in Tinker Salas 2015, 134.

45. Coronil and Skurski 1991.

46. López Maya 2002. This figure does not include labor protests or strikes.

47. Wilpert 2007.

48. Martinez, Fox, and Farrell 2010.

49. Wilpert 2007.

50. Kozloff 2005.

51. Wilpert 2007.

52. Weisbrot, Ray, and Sandoval 2009. This figure represents real social spending across this period (adjusted for inflation).

53. See, e.g., Clara Han's ethnography *Life in Debt: Times of Care and Violence in Neoliberal Chile* (2012).

54. Kirk 2015. Cuban medical professionals worked in Venezuela on renewable two-year contracts, and Venezuela sold petroleum to Cuba at preferential rates. The Cuban government has been sending its doctors abroad on medical aid missions for over fifty years, though historically on a much smaller scale than reflected by the number of doctors working in Barrio Adentro (Feinsilver 2008). In fact, so many of Cuba's doctors worked in Venezuela in the mid-2000s that a number of neighborhood clinics in Cuba closed, leading to discontent and resentment among Cubans accustomed to the family doctor model (Brotherton 2012).

55. See Kirk 2015.

56. Alvarado et al. 2008; Weisbrot, Ray, and Sandoval 2009; Westhoff et al. 2010.

57. Palmer 2003; Waitzkin et al. 2001; Zulawski 2007.

58. Hellinger 2011, 43.

59. Kirk 2015.

60. PROVEA 2007; BBC News 2005; Briggs and Mantini-Briggs 2009.

61. Arsenault 2013.

62. Armada et al. 2009.

63. Armada et al. 2009.

64. Kirk 2015.

65. Armada et al. 2009, 171. The country's population in 2005 was approximately 27 million.

66. Sen 2002.

67. Izquierdo 2005.

68. Izquierdo 2005, 768.

69. Many examples of culturally specific notions of health may be found in the anthropological literature, e.g., Naomi Adelson's ethnography of the Cree conception of "being alive well," which includes hunting, eating certain foods, and maintaining proper relationships (Adelson 2000).

70. UNICEF 2014.

71. UNICEF 2014.

72. Wilpert 2011; United Nations 2015.

73. ECLAC 2015.

74. UNDP 2010.

75. UNDP 2010.

76. UNDP 2010.

77. PAHO 2012.

78. The city has five municipalities. Libertador is the historical and political center and is the seat of the national government, most of the ministries, and Miraflores, the Presidential Palace. It is home to many of the city's barrios.

79. INE 2002.

80. Fernandes 2010; Velasco 2015; Schiller 2018; Smilde and Hellinger 2011.

81. Fernandes 2007, 2010; Martinez, Fox, and Farrell 2010; Schiller 2018.

82. I received permission to conduct research from the Municipal Health Department of Libertador, the local council (*junta parroquial*) of Santa Teresa, and the Health Committee (Comité de Salud) of the main Barrio Adentro clinic in Santa Teresa. In Caracas I was formally affiliated with the Center for Advanced Studies and the Centro de Antropología at the Instituto Venezolano de Investigaciones Científicas (IVIC). The University of Chicago Social and Behavioral Sciences Institutional Review Board approved this research.

83. I also found, as the sociologist David Smilde asserts, that "many of the middle and upper classes have never in their lives set foot in a popular *barrio*" (Smilde 2008).

84. U.S. Department of State n.d.

85. Interactions with Cuban medical workers were somewhat different. They knew they were under scrutiny by people who disapproved of their presence. When

I began research in 2006, the Cuban Medical Mission was not allowing doctors to speak to foreign visitors. This changed by 2008, when Cuban doctors invited me to observe and participate in the daily life of their clinics. Still, I sensed that they felt they had to tread carefully in Venezuela, which was confirmed one night when a Cuban friend interrupted a conversation about her work in Caracas's barrios to ask me if there was any possibility my apartment had been bugged.

86. Salter and Weltman 2011.
87. Samet and Schiller 2017.

CHAPTER TWO

1. Biomedicine and religion are often intertwined, though biomedicine often presents itself as a purely secular endeavor. See, for example, the special issue of the journal *Medical Anthropology* titled "Nonsecular Medical Anthropology" (Whitmarsh and Roberts 2016).

2. For more detailed discussion of José Gregorio Hernández, see Ferrándiz 1998; Margolies 1984; Low 1988. María Lionza is an indigenous religious figure and the central player in the country's syncretic religious tradition known as *espiritismo,* or the cult of María Lionza. In a famous statue of her that looms over drivers on a major Caracas highway, María Lionza looks strong and powerful, riding a wild tapir naked and holding a female pelvis to symbolize fertility.

3. Margolies 1984, 29.

4. Margolies 1984, 29.

5. Ferrándiz 1998; Friedmann 1966.

6. Neuman 2014. People often complained that the Vatican was dragging its feet on José Gregorio's canonization in spite of overwhelming evidence.

7. Mara Gomez, director of Libertador Municipality health department, personal communication, Caracas, November 14, 2008.

8. Research participants commonly complained that the international news media presented a one-sided perspective of the Chávez administration's policies by failing to focus on government social policies aimed to reduce social inequalities. Media analysis supports this claim (Salter and Weltman 2011).

9. Briggs and Mantini-Briggs 2009; Mara Gomez, personal communication, Caracas, November 14, 2008.

10. Cooper 2015.

CHAPTER THREE

1. Ochoa 2014.

2. Exceptions to the pattern of responses I describe in this chapter included a small number of patients who before the advent of Barrio Adentro developed long-

term, personalized relationships with specific doctors in public hospitals and who were able to mobilize access to care and services from these physicians. Another exception to this pattern involved a few patients I met who used Barrio Adentro but expressed a preference for Venezuelan or other non-Cuban doctors. They questioned Cuban doctors' technical competence, concerned that medical training and practice in Cuba operated with outdated technologies and insufficient levels of technical specialization.

3. Nations and Rebhun 1988; Taussig 1980; West 1984.

4. Auyero 2012; Briggs and Mantini-Briggs 2003; Maternowska 2006; Nations and Rebhun 1988; Roberts 2012a, 2012b; Scheper-Hughes 1993.

5. Nations and Rebhun 1988, 29.

6. Crandon-Malamud 1991; Waitzkin 1991.

7. Andaya 2009; Brotherton 2012.

8. Bernstein 2013; Whiteford and Branch 2008.

9. Briggs and Mantini-Briggs 2009.

10. Perez 2008, 229, 232.

11. Foucault 1975.

12. Davenport 2000, 311.

13. Prentice 2012; Davenport 2000; Bernstein 2013.

14. Bernstein 2013; Davenport 2000.

15. Bernstein 2013, 166.

16. Bernstein 2013, 167.

17. Farquhar 1994; Kirmayer 2004; Van Dongen and Elema 2001.

18. Coordinación Nacional de Barrio Adentro 2008.

19. PROVEA 2007.

20. Antze and Lambek 1996; Cartwright 2007; Cole 2001; High 2009.

21. Medical anthropologists describe how patients from socially and politically marginalized groups in other places, including indigenous Maya and Inuit patients, similarly interpreted interactions with medical professionals as continuations of a longer history of marginalization and exclusion from nation-state belonging (Berry 2008; Browne 2007; O'Neil 1989).

22. Farquhar 1994; Mol 2008; Yates-Doerr 2012.

23. Béhague 2002; Béhague et al. 2002; Crandon 1986; Roberts 2012a, 2012b; Waitzkin 1991.

24. Roberts 2012a, 88.

CHAPTER FOUR

1. "Popular medicine" is the term I use in this book, but similar terms include complementary and alternative medicine.

2. Cant and Sharma 2014; Baer 2015. For simplicity, this discussion presents biomedicine and other healing systems as separate entities, although different healing systems commonly interact and borrow from one another.

3. Baer 2015.

4. Cant and Sharma 2014.

5. The anthropologist Hans Baer defines biomedical hegemony in a pluralistic medical setting as a "dominative medical system" to emphasize that healing traditions coexist in patterned, unequal relations to each other (Baer 2011).

6. Starr 1982; Cueto and Palmer 2015. In addition to working with state officials to establish formal legal frameworks granting biomedicine privileged (in some cases exclusive) rights to practice medicine, proponents of biomedicine attempted to shape cultural beliefs. The anthropologist and physician Dan Blumhagen analyzed the history of the doctor's white coat, noting that biomedical doctors proactively organized to make the white lab coat a central part of their identities in order to win more authority and respect for their profession by associating themselves with laboratory science (Blumhagen 1979).

7. Kleinman 1997.

8. For an overview of this history, see Cueto and Palmer 2015. Doctors have played an outsized role in Latin American politics compared to other regions of the world. Strengthening biomedicine's authority was one goal among many. The most famous physicians in Latin American politics, Ché Guevara and Salvador Allende, focused on expanding health care access to the poor.

9. Baer 2011; Brotherton 2012.

10. Also worth noting is the fact that Barrio Adentro primary care clinics did not maintain patient charts (except for records of infant immunizations). Patients maintained their own records (mostly test results) that they brought with them to doctors' visits. As scholars have noted for other countries, this practice increases patient control over their diagnoses and treatments (though with potential loss of continuity of care; Nunley 1988).

11. Carroll 2010.

12. Brotherton 2008, 2012.

13. Westhoff et al. 2010, 521. Pharmaceuticals provided in Barrio Adentro community clinics were Cuban-produced generics. The government gave away non-Cuban drugs (generics and brand-name) through other programs.

14. Based on a joint Ministry of Health and pharmaceutical industry study (Marcano 2008).

15. I observed many more medical encounters in Barrio Adentro clinics. This number reflects the number of office visits for which I took detailed, structured notes on the interactions, including reason for the visit, topics discussed, demographic background of patients, and the outcome of the encounter (i.e., treatments, advice given).

16. E.M.S. 2008.

17. Johnson 2009.

18. This claim applies to research participants who were majority poor and working-class Caraqueños. I cannot say whether wealthier Venezuelans would also agree with this claim.

19. Starting in the mid-twentieth century, the cult of María Lionza, which had been practiced by rural peasant populations southwest of Caracas (Yaracuy State), expanded to cities and came to be widely practiced by people from a range of social classes, although its centers of practice were usually based in barrios. For ethnographic accounts of the cult of Maria Lionza, see Ferrándiz 1998, 2004; Pollak-Eltz 1982; Taussig 1997.

20. The anthropologist Angelina Pollak-Eltz explained that at the end of the 1800s wealthy Venezuelans practiced spiritism as popularized by Allan Kardec; the practice later entered popular religious and healing cultures (Pollak-Eltz 1982).

21. Pollak-Eltz 1982; Kay Scaramelli, personal communication, Jan. 18, 2009; Paullier 2011.

22. Ferrándiz 1998; Fernandes 2010.

23. Ferrándiz 1998, 46–47.

24. Pollak-Eltz 1982, 28–29.

25. Popular healing products included dried herbs and plants, pills, baths, soaps, colognes, candles, religious figures, books, and a variety of other objects for use in espiritismo, santería, New Age and Asian-inspired healing, cults of saints like José Gregorio Hernández, and herbal and botanical medicine.

26. National Public Radio 2007; Associated Press 2008, Brassesco 2008. Some journalists and research participants claimed that *santería*'s popularity was directly related to Cuban medical workers in Barrio Adentro who were popularizing the practice among local residents.

27. This logic underlines a 2017 story in National Geographic titled, "In Need of a Cure: Venezuelans Are Turning to Faith Healers as the Nation's Health Care Crisis Deepens" (Kohut 2017). The story reports on desperately sick people, unable to access biomedical treatments, who seek out spiritist healers and pray to José Gregorio (see the conclusion for a discussion of Venezuela's economic crisis since 2013 and its effects on health care). The story implies that if people had access to biomedicine they would not use popular medicine because of its evident inferiority.

28. Ferrándiz 1998, 39; Palmer 2003; Sowell 2001.

29. Ferrándiz 1988, 2004; Glenn 2009; Margolies 1984; Low 1988. One example is the explanation anthropologists give for the emergence of the cult of devotion to the popular saint José Gregorio Hernández. As Setha Low explained, "The rise of Hernandez's cult . . . can be interpreted as a response to the turmoil and sociopolitical upheaval that began in Venezuela in the 1940s" (Low 1988, 149).

30. Martinez, Fox, and Farrell 2010; Fernandes 2010; Valencia 2015.

31. UNDP 2010. Based on polling data, subjective assessments of quality of life among Venezuelans were among the highest in the world during this period. According to Gallup's Global Wellbeing Survey of 2010, Venezuela ranked sixth out of 124 countries in a poll measuring subjective assessments of one's quality of life (Boothroyd 2010): "64% of Venezuelans considered themselves to be 'thriving' [ranking their current lives 7 or above and future lives 8 or above on a scale of 1–10]. . . . Beaten only by Denmark (79%), Canada (69%), Sweden (69%), and

Australia (66%), and scoring the same levels of 'thriving' as Finland, Venezuela occupied the highest position in those countries considered to be in the 'developing world' and came first out of all the Latin American nations" (Boothroyd 2010; see also Gallup 2010).

32. Wilpert 2011; UNDP 2015; ECLAC 2015.

33. Farquhar 2002, 28. See also Farquhar and Zhang 2005, 2012.

34. Bolivarian Republic of Venezuela 1999.

35. Bolivarian Republic of Venezuela 1999.

36. Gobierno Bolivariana de Venezuela 2001.

37. Reporte 2008.

38. Cueto and Palmer 2015; Torri 2010; Mignone et al. 2007. Although there are some parallels between practices of intercultural health and what the Venezuelan government was doing, I did not observe anyone use this term during fieldwork.

39. Perez 2008, 79.

40. Feinsilver 1993, 40. However, as Perez and others have shown, Cuban doctors were not uncaring state agents whose primary concern was coercing patients into biomedical submission. A deeply felt humanism animated the work of many Cuban medical professionals, existing in concert with government efforts to optimize national health indicators by carefully managing individual health practices. For a nuanced ethnographic account of how Cuban doctors negotiate everyday tensions of managing population health, see Elise Andaya's book, *Conceiving Cuba: Women, Reproduction, and the State in the Post-Soviet Era* (Andaya 2014). Andaya found that doctors became intimately involved in patients' prenatal care and sometimes reprimanded families of women with high-risk pregnancies for not encouraging enough rest, for example. Her work also reveals that doctors and nurses cared deeply about their patients and expressed that care through acts of nurturance, which patients appreciated and reciprocated, sometimes in the form of gifts.

41. Based on my participant observation conducted in 2006, 2008, and early 2009. The exception was for infants; nurses kept records of their check-ups and immunization schedules.

42. WHO 2001.

43. Brotherton 2008, 270.

44. Brotherton 2008.

CHAPTER FIVE

1. Participation in community health activism and elderly exercise clubs was highly gendered, with women making up the vast majority of people involved in both activities. In Bolivarian Venezuela women participated heavily in government-sponsored community social programs, comprising up to 90 percent of participants in some cases (Fernandes 2007). Community health activism in other Latin American countries, such as Chile and Nicaragua, involves mostly women (Paley 2001; Nading 2014). Scholars suggest that in the case of community activism, this gen-

dered dynamic reflects understandings of women as the traditional caregivers for the family and in the community (see Schiller 2018). The preponderance of women in these organizations could also reflect a response to the Chávez government explicitly encouraging women to participate more fully in politics, given their relative exclusion from this arena in the past (Fernandes 2007). Why the exercise clubs mostly comprised women is less clearly related to ideologies of women as nurturers or a history of gender inequality in politics. However, this finding was in keeping with my observation of a gender difference in health care seeking more generally, with more women than men seeking care in Barrio Adentro clinics.

2. Smilde and Hellinger 2011; Martinez et al. 2010; Fernandes 2010; Schiller 2009.

3. Armada et al. 2009; Alvarado et al. 2008.

4. Hellinger 2011, 55.

5. Joropo is a popular style of Venezuelan folk music and dancing.

6. In 2009 a club in Argentina celebrated the thirty-second anniversary of its founding, and one club recently featured in a local Chilean newspaper was founded in 1984. At least one Grandparents Club was founded in Caracas in 1997, more than five years before the government began promoting them nationwide (*El Universal* 2005). Clubs for older adults also exist in many other Latin American countries and in Spain and Portugal (and in other settings, including North America).

7. Garcia 2009.

8. The phrase "encerarrse in la casa" refers also to a sense of inseguridad related to the widespread and intensely felt fear of crime in Caracas.

9. Mahmood 2005; Bourdieu 1977.

10. Hahrie Han documents a similar process of engagement in political activism among underprivileged North Americans (Han 2009).

11. The widely held conviction among members that participation in Grandparents Clubs led to better personal health mirrors findings by at least one formal study of a Grandparents Club in Cuba, in which researchers found participation led to improvements in blood pressure, walking, general fitness, and psychological well-being and reductions in joint pain, obesity, and reliance on pharmaceuticals (Morales and Acosta 1991).

12. The Third Age (*la tercera edad*) is a term used cross-culturally to refer to the stage of life following retirement (for those in formal employment) and the lessening of responsibility for parenting one's own children (many older adults who belonged to the Third Age in Santa Teresa continued to care for grandchildren, sometimes full-time).

13. López Maya, Smilde, and Stephany 2006; López Maya 2002.

14. López Maya 2002, 211.

15. PROVEA 2011.

16. El Informador 2009.

17. Huenchuan 2009.

18. A free trip to Cuba for a week, co-sponsored by Venezuela and Cuba, was the most exciting state-sponsored activity of the Grandparents Club.

19. In contrast, I never saw medical workers wearing clothes suggestive of political affiliation. Medical workers exclusively wore unmarked street clothes and white coats.

20. Scholars often contrast participatory democracy with representative democracy, in which ordinary people rely on elected representatives to conduct the affairs of government.

21. The concept of community participation in health has a decades-long history in international public health circles, where it has been celebrated as a low-cost way to improve people's health and empower local actors. In the 1980s and 1990s many Latin American governments developed cadres of community health workers to advance national public health goals. These programs were often established as part of neoliberal reforms that cut public spending and devolved responsibility for health care onto individuals and local communities (see Cooper 2015 for a discussion of how Barrio Adentro community health workers' experiences differed from this earlier generation of community health workers in the region).

22. MSDS n.d.

CHAPTER SIX

1. Simón Pineda, president of Fundación José Felix Ribas, personal communication, 2006.

2. I heard three reports from residents about murders during my fieldwork in 2008–9. Of these, two were said to have occurred in Plaza la Concordia and one was the murder of a pharmacist during an armed robbery in his shop.

3. Chávez Morales 2008.

4. Chávez Morales 2008, 39.

5. Sarmiendo Garmendia 2008, 3.

6. Sarmiendo Garmendia 2008, 3.

7. Maribel Navas 2008, 8.

8. Maribel Navas 2008, 8.

9. Venezuela Analysis 2006.

10. Venezuela Analysis 2006.

11. Agencia Venezolana de Noticias 2016.

12. Venezuela Analysis 2006.

13. Hopper 2003; Garcia 2010; Bourgois and Schonberg 2009; Desjarlais 1997; Luhrmann 2008, 2009; Estroff 1985.

14. Media reports on the ten-year anniversary of the Negra Hipólita program said that as of 2016, thirty-seven long-term rehabilitation centers were operating nationwide (Agencia Venezolana de Noticias 2016).

15. For example, a 2004 document that Hugo Chávez delivered to the United Nations was titled, "We Want to End Poverty? Let's Give Power to the Poor" (Chávez Frias 2004). Also distributed as a pamphlet in Venezuela, the paper argued that state education, health, and nutrition programs enabled poor people to empower themselves.

16. For example, the Pan American Health Organization published an evaluation of primary health services in Venezuela in 2006 titled *Barrio Adentro: The Right to Health and Social Inclusion in Venezuela* (OPS 2006). The report described clinics in poor neighborhoods as promoting empowerment and social inclusion for marginalized residents.

17. One Negra Hipólita center director explicitly linked rehabilitation with citizenship in an interview with a journalist, describing the people living in his center as "an army that one day was destroying this city and today they are working in building. We are an example of good citizens" (Agencia Venezolana de Noticias 2016).

18. Weddle 2016.

19. Douglas 1970, 115.

20. Douglas 1970, 117.

21. Žižek 1993, 202.

22. Žižek 1993, 203.

CONCLUSION

1. Good and DelVecchio Good 1993.

2. There are striking parallels between the practices that I observed as meaningful for Venezuelan patients, medical workers, and medical students and what Claire Wendland describes in her ethnography of Malawian medicine, *A Heart for the Work: Journeys through an African Medical School* (Wendland 2010). Wendland, a medical anthropologist and obstetrician from the United States, found that medical students and medical workers in Malawi understood their work as motivated by and expressing "*love, heart, passion,* or *spirit,*" which they saw as more important to the practice of medicine than objectivity or technical competence (Wendland 2010, 177–78; original emphasis). She contrasted this emotional orientation to medicine with norms in the Global North, saying, "In the United States, I have often heard students, residents, and practicing physicians say of a colleague, 'He may be an asshole, but he's a really good doc.' I never heard anything similar in Malawi and have come to believe that it would be heard as nonsensical there. The work itself, for these students, required heart" (178).

3. Stigma associated with using government health care in the United States applies to Medicaid users more than Medicare users, as Medicaid serves people with limited income while Medicare is for people over age sixty-five who paid into the system during their working years via payroll taxes.

4. Conversations with past research participants occurred via email in fall 2017. Academic analyses of the current situation include those found in María et al. 2017; Grandin 2017; Hetland and Cicciarello-Maher 2017; Cicciarello-Maher 2017; Fernandes 2017; Stefanoni 2017; Hellinger 2016b; Smilde 2016; Hetland 2017, 2016; Ellner and Koerner 2016a, 2016b.

5. See Telesur 2017 for details of each death.

6. For simplicity's sake, I present the political situation in broad brushstrokes. But Venezuelan politics is far more complicated than a two-party system of pro- and anti-government supporters. Many factions exist within these groups and others operate outside this binary, such as Marea Socialista (Socialist Tide), whose members openly criticize the Maduro government and call for deepening socialism in line with Chávez's vision.

7. Kohut 2017; PBS NewsHour 2017; Keane 2016; Casey 2016.

8. Pestano 2017.

9. Koerner 2017.

10. Strange 2017.

11. Pestano 2016.

12. Ethnographies of revolution include Lancaster 1994; Shah 2014; Earle and Simonelli 2005; Lan 1985; Pettigrew 2013; Wolf 1969; Donham 1999; Schiekle 2015; Scott 1976.

13. For this definition I draw on the anthropologist Bjørn Thomassen's conditions comprising political revolution in his article "Notes Toward an Anthropology of Political Revolutions" (2012, 683–84).

14. As Thomassen notes, "Revolutions more than any other event in modern history represent . . . moments where given hierarchies, social norms, and shared values are brought into question" (2012, 701).

15. Shah 2014, 339.

REFERENCES

Adelson, Naomi. 2000. *"Being Alive Well": Health and the Politics of Cree Well-Being.* Toronto: University of Toronto Press.

Agencia Venezolana de Noticias (AVN). 2016. "Mission Negra Hipolita Celebrates 10 Years Providing Solidarity to Destitute People." January 14. www.avn.info.ve /contenido/mission-negra-hipolita-celebrates-10-years-providing-solidarity-destitute-people. Accessed February 7, 2017.

Alvarado, Carlos H., María E. Martínez, Sarai Vivas-Martínez, Nuramy J. Gutiérrez, and Wolfram Metzger. 2008. "Social Change and Health Policy in Venezuela." *Social Medicine* 3 (2): 95–109.

Andaya, Elise. 2009. "The Gift of Health: Socialist Medical Practice and Shifting Material and Moral Economies in Post-Soviet Cuba." *Medical Anthropology Quarterly* 23 (4): 357–74.

———. 2014. *Conceiving Cuba: Reproduction, Women, and the State in the Post-Soviet Era.* New Brunswick, NJ: Rutgers University Press.

Antze, Paul, and Michael Lambek. 1996. *Tense Past: Cultural Essays in Trauma and Memory.* New York: Routledge.

Armada, Francisco, Carles Muntaner, Haejoo Chung, Leslie Williams-Brennan, and Joan Benach. 2009. "Barrio Adentro and the Reduction of Health Inequalities in Venezuela: An Appraisal of the First Years." *International Journal of Health Services* 39 (1): 161–87.

Arsenault, Chris. 2013. "Clinics Attacked in Venezuela Vote Violence." *Al Jazeera America,* April 17. www.aljazeera.com/indepth/features/2013/04/2013417716285301 .html. Accessed February 22, 2015.

Associated Press. 2008. "Venezuelans Increasingly Turn to Santería." February 8. www.msnbc.msn.com/id/23057224/ns/world_news-venezuela/t/venezuelans-increasingly-turn-santeria/#.TkowL79r390. Accessed August 16, 2011.

Auyero, Javier. 2012. *Patients of the State: The Politics of Waiting in Argentina.* Durham, NC: Duke University Press.

Baer, Hans A. 2011. "Medical Pluralism: An Evolving and Contested Concept in Medical Anthropology." In *A Companion to Medical Anthropology,* edited by Merrill Singer and Pamela I. Erickson, 405–24. Malden, MA: Wiley-Blackwell.

BBC News. 2005. "Venezuela Medics March over Jobs." July 15. http://news.bbc.co.uk/2/hi/4688117.stm. Accessed February 22, 2015.

———. 2016. "Venezuela Military to Distribute Medicine to Hospitals." November 3. www.bbc.com/news/world-latin-america-37859183. Accessed April 19, 2017.

Béhague, Dominique. 2002. "Beyond the Simple Economics of Cesarean Section Birthing: Women's Resistance to Social Inequality." *Culture, Medicine, and Psychiatry* 26 (4): 473–507.

Béhague, Dominique, Cesar Victoria, and Fernando Barros. 2002. "Consumer Demand for Caesarean Sections in Brazil: Informed Decision Making, Patient Choice, or Social Inequality? A Population Based Birth Cohort Study Linking Ethnographic and Epidemiological Methods." *The BMJ* 324: 942.

Bernstein, Alyssa. 2013. "Transformative Medical Education and the Making of New Clinical Subjectivities through Cuban-Bolivian Medical Diplomacy." In *Health Travels: Cuban Health(care) On and Off the Island,* edited by Nancy J. Burke, 154–77. Berkeley: University of California Medical Humanities Press.

Berry, Nicole. 2008. "Who's Judging the Quality of Care? Indigenous Maya and the Problem of 'Not Being Attended.'" *Medical Anthropology* 27 (2): 164–89.

———. 2012. *Unsafe Motherhood: Mayan Maternal Mortality and Subjectivity in Post-War Guatemala.* New York: Berghahn Books.

Blumhagen, Dan. 1979. "The Doctor's White Coat: The Image of the Physician in Modern America." *Annals of Internal Medicine* 91 (1): 111–16.

Bolivarian Republic of Venezuela. 1999. *Constitution of the Bolivarian Republic of Venezuela.* Caracas.

Boothroyd, Rachael. 2011. "Venezuela Comes Sixth in Gallup 'Wellbeing' Survey." April 24. Venezuelanalysis.com, http://venezuelanalysis.com/news/6149. Accessed November 28, 2018.

Boothroyd-Rojas, Rachael, and Lucas Koerner. 2016. "Community-Delivered Food, Clean Clinics, and Queue-Less Banks: A Glimpse into VA's Week in Venezuela." *Venezuela Analysis,* December 10. https://venezuelanalysis.com/analysis/12827. Accessed April 19, 2017.

Bourgois, Phillipe, and Jeff Schonberg. 2009. *Righteous Dopefiend.* Berkeley: University of California Press.

Brassesco, Javier. 2008. "La santería vive un auge inusitado." *El Universal,* September 30, 3–1.

Briggs, Charles, and Clara Mantini-Briggs. 2003. *Stories in the Time of Cholera: Racial Profiling during a Medical Nightmare.* Berkeley: University of California Press.

———. 2009. "Confronting Health Disparities: Latin American Social Medicine in Venezuela." *American Journal of Public Health* 99 (3): 549–55.

———. 2016. *Tell Me Why My Children Died: Rabies, Indigenous Knowledge, and Communicative Justice.* Durham, NC: Duke University Press.

Brotherton, P. Sean. 2008. "We Have to Think Like Capitalists but Continue Being Socialists: Medicalized Subjectivities, Emergent Capital, and Socialist Entrepreneurs in Post-Soviet Cuba." *American Ethnologist* 35 (2): 259–74.

———. 2012. *Revolutionary Medicine: Health and the Body in Post-Socialist Cuba.* Durham, NC: Duke University Press.

Brown, Wendy. 2015. *Undoing the Demos: Neoliberalism's Stealth Revolution.* New York: Zone Books.

Browne, Annette. 2007. "Clinical Encounters between Nurses and First Nations Women in a Western Canadian Hospital." *Social Science and Medicine* 64 (10): 2165–76.

Butt, Leslie. 2002. "The Suffering Stranger: Medical Anthropology and International Morality." *Medical Anthropology: Cross-Cultural Studies in Health and Illness* 21 (1): 1–24.

Cant, Sarah, and Ursula Sharma. 2014. *A New Medical Pluralism? Alternative Medicine, Doctors, Patients and the State.* London: Routledge.

Carroll, Rory. 2010. "Hugo Chávez's Twitter Habit Proves a Popular Success." *Guardian,* August 10. www.guardian.co.uk/world/2010/aug/10/hugo-chavez-twitter-venezuela#_jmpo_. Accessed March 7, 2012.

Cartwright, Elizabeth. 2007. "Bodily Remembering: Memory, Place, and Understanding Latino Folk Illnesses among the Amuzgos Indians of Oaxaca, Mexico." *Culture, Medicine, and Psychiatry* 31 (4): 527–45.

Casey, Nicholas. 2016. "Dying Infants and No Medicine: Inside Venezuela's Failing Hospitals." *New York Times,* May 15. www.nytimes.com/2016/05/16/world/americas/dying-infants-and-no-medicine-inside-venezuelas-failing-hospitals.html. Accessed April 19, 2017.

Chávez Frias, Hugo. 2004. "¿Queremos acabar con la pobreza? Demos poder a los pobres (la experiencia venezolana)." United Nations, September. Reunión de Jefes de Estado Convocada por el Presidente de Brasil Luiz Inácio Lula da Silva.

Chávez Morales, Jorge. 2008. "Cuatro 'piedras' por el cobre: Recicladores de metales entregan hierramientes a indigentes para que roban obras de arte, barandas de puente y cables y les pagan con drogas." *Últimas Noticias (Caracas),* February 24, 3.

Cicciarello-Maher, George. 2013. *We Created Chávez: A People's History of the Venezuelan Revolution.* Durham, NC: Duke University Press.

———. 2017. "Which Way out of the Venezuelan Crisis?" *Jacobin,* July 29. https://jacobinmag.com/2017/07/venezuela-elections-chavez-maduro-bolivarianism. Accessed November 8, 2017.

Cole, Jennifer. 2001. *Forget Colonialism? Sacrifice and the Art of Memory in Madagascar.* Berkeley: University of California Press.

Cooper, Amy. 2015. "What Does Health Activism Mean in Venezuela's Barrio Adentro Program? Understanding Community Health Work in Political and Cultural Context." *Annals of Anthropological Practice* 39 (1): 58–72.

———. 2017. "Moving Medicine inside the Neighborhood: Health Care and Sociospatial Transformation in Caracas, Venezuela." *Medicine Anthropology Theory* 4 (1): 20–45.

Cooper, Amy, Robert Samet, and Naomi Schiller, eds. 2015. "Protests and Polarization in Venezuela after Chávez." Hot Spots, *Cultural Anthropology* website, February 5. https://culanth.org/fieldsights/630-protests-and-polarization-in-venezuela-after-chavez. Accessed April 30, 2017.

Coordinación Nacional de Barrio Adentro. 2008. *Barrio Adentro: Una obra de corazón*. Caracas: Ministerio del Poder Popular para la Comunicación y la Información.

Coronil, Fernando. 1997. *The Magical State: Nature, Money, and Modernity in Venezuela*. Chicago: University of Chicago Press.

Coronil, Fernando, and Julie Skurski. 1991. "Dismembering and Remembering the Nation: The Semantics of Political Violence in Venezuela." *Comparative Studies in Society and History* 33 (2): 288–337.

Crandon, Libbet. 1986. "Medical Dialogue and the Political Economy of Medical Pluralism: A Case from Rural Highland Bolivia." *American Ethnologist* 13 (3): 463–76.

Crandon-Malamud, Libbet. 1991. *From the Fat of Our Souls: Social Change, Political Process, and Medical Pluralism in Bolivia*. Berkeley: University of California Press.

Cueto, Marcos, and Steven Palmer. 2015. *Medicine and Public Health in Latin America: A History*. Cambridge: Cambridge University Press.

Davenport, Beverly Ann. 2000. "Witnessing and the Medical Gaze: How Medical Students Learn to See at a Free Clinic for the Homeless." *Medical Anthropology Quarterly* 14 (3): 310–27.

Desjarlais, Robert. 1997. *Shelter Blues: Sanity and Selfhood among the Homeless*. Philadelphia: University of Pennsylvania Press.

Donham, Donald D. 1999. *Marxist Modern: An Ethnographic History of the Ethiopian Revolution*. Berkeley: University of California Press.

Douglas, Mary. [1966] 1970. *Purity and Danger: An Analysis of the Concepts of Pollution and Taboo*. London: Penguin.

Earle, Duncan, and Jeanne Simonelli. 2005. *Uprising of Hope: Sharing the Zapatista Journey to Alternative Development*. Walnut Creek, CA: Altamira Press.

Economic Commission for Latin America and the Caribbean (ECLAC). 2015. *Statistical Yearbook of Latin America and the Caribbean*. Santiago, Chile: United Nations.

Edmonds, Alexander. 2012. "A Right to Beauty." *Anthropology Now* 4 (1): 3–9.

Ellner, Steve. 2008. *Rethinking Venezuelan Politics: Class, Conflict, and the Chávez Phenomenon*. Boulder: Lynne Rienner Publishers.

Ellner, Steve, and Lucas Koerner. 2016a. "Steve Ellner: Democratization of PSUV Is Key to Chavismo's Future." *Venezuela Analysis,* October 10. https://venezuelanalysis.com/analysis/12716. Accessed April 19, 2017.

———. 2016b. "Steve Ellner Part II: Is the Bolivarian Revolution a Populist Failure?" *Venezuela Analysis,* October 17. https://venezuelanalysis.com/analysis/12723. Accessed April 19, 2017.

Ellner, Steve, and Miguel Tinker Salas. 2005. "Introduction: The Venezuelan Exceptionalism Thesis: Separating Myth from Reality." *Latin American Perspectives* 32 (2): 5–19.

E.M.S. 2008. "Venta de medicamentos reportó aumento de 10.11% en 2007." *El Nacional,* February 1.

Estroff, Sue. 1985. *Making it Crazy: An Ethnography of Psychiatric Clients in an American Community.* Berkeley: University of California Press.

Farquhar, Judith. 1994. "Eating Chinese Medicine." *Cultural Anthropology* 9 (4): 471–97.

———. 2002. *Appetites: Food and Sex in Post-Socialist China.* Durham, NC: Duke University Press.

Farquhar, Judith, and Qicheng Zhang. 2005. "Biopolitical Beijing: Pleasure, Sovereignty, and Self-Cultivation in China's Capital." *Cultural Anthropology* 20 (3): 303–27.

———. 2012. *Ten Thousand Things: Nurturing Life in Contemporary Beijing.* New York: Zone Books.

Feinsilver, Julie. 1993. *Healing the Masses: Cuban Health Politics at Home and Abroad.* Berkeley: University of California Press.

———. 2008. "Oil-for-Doctors: Cuban Medical Diplomacy Gets a Little Help from a Venezuelan Friend." *Nueva Sociedad* 216: 107–22.

Fernandes, Sujatha. 2007. "Barrio Women and Popular Politics in Chávez's Venezuela." *Latin American Politics and Society* 49 (3): 97–127.

———. 2010. *Who Can Stop the Drums? Urban Social Movements in Chávez's Venezuela.* Durham, NC: Duke University Press.

———. 2017. "What's Left of the Bolivarian Revolution?" *NACLA,* July 26. https://nacla.org/news/2017/07/27/what%e2%80%99s-left-bolivarian-revolution. Accessed November 8, 2017.

Ferrándiz, Francisco. 1998. "José Gregorio Hernández: A Chameleonic Presence in the Eye of the Medical Hurricane." *Kroeber Anthropological Society Papers* 83: 37–56.

———. 2004. "The Body as Wound: Possession, Malandros, and Everyday Violence in Venezuela." *Critique of Anthropology* 24: 107–33.

Fischer, Edward. 2014. *The Good Life: Aspiration, Dignity, and the Anthropology of Wellbeing.* Stanford, CA: Stanford University Press.

Foucault, Michel. 1975. *The Birth of the Clinic: An Archaeology of Medical Perception.* New York: Vintage.

———. 1977. *Discipline and Punish: The Birth of the Prison.* New York: Vintage.

———. 1980. *The History of Sexuality, Vol. 1: An Introduction.* New York: Vintage.

Fox News. 2016. "Venezuela's Health Care Is Such a Failure, Scraped Knee Turns into Medical Crisis." October 4. www.foxnews.com/health/2016/10/04/venezuela-health-care-is-such-failure-scraped-knee-turns-into-medical-crisis.html. Accessed April 19, 2017.

Fraser, Gertrude. 1998. *African-American Midwifery in the South: Dialogues of Birth, Race, and Memory.* Cambridge, MA: Harvard University Press.

Friedmann, John. 1966. *Regional Development Policy: A Case Study of Venezuela.* Cambridge, MA: MIT Press.

Gallup Organization. 2010. *Global Wellbeing: Who's Thriving Worldwide.* www .gallup.com/poll/126977/global-wellbeing-surveys-find-nations-worlds-apart. aspx. Accessed June 13, 2011.

Ganti, Tejaswini. 2014. "Neoliberalism." *Annual Review of Anthropology* 43: 89–104.

Garcia, Angela. 2010. *The Pastoral Clinic: Addiction and Dispossession Along the Rio Grande.* Berkeley: University of California Press.

Garcia Quiñones, Rolando. 2009. "Social Policies, Family Arrangements, and Population Ageing in Cuba." Paper presented at International Seminar on Family Support Networks and Population Ageing (United Nations Population Fund), June 3–4, Doha, Qatar.

Georges, Eugenia. 2008. *Bodies of Knowledge: The Medicalization of Reproduction in Greece.* Nashville, TN: Vanderbilt University Press.

Glenn, Wade. 2009. "Traditional Medicine for the Ills of Modernity: The Cult of Maria Lionza in Venezuela." Paper presented at the American Anthropological Association 108th Annual Meeting, Philadelphia, December 6.

Glick, Leonard. 1967. "Medicine as an Ethnographic Category: The Gimi of the New Guinea Highlands." *Ethnology* 6 (1): 31–56.

Gobierno Bolivariana de Venezuela. 2001. *Gaceta Oficial de la República Bolivariana de Venezuela No. 37135.* February 6, Caracas.

Good, Byron J., and Mary-Jo DelVecchio Good. 1993. "Learning Medicine: The Constructing of Medical Knowledge at Harvard Medical School." In *Knowledge, Power and Practice: The Anthropology of Medicine and Everyday Life,* 81–107. Berkeley: University of California Press.

Grandin, Greg. 2017. "What Is to Be Done in Venezuela?" *The Nation,* May 1. www .thenation.com/article/what-is-to-be-done-in-venezuela/. Accessed November 8, 2017.

Halliburton, Murphy. 2003. "The Importance of a Pleasant Process of Treatment: Lessons on Healing from South India." *Culture, Medicine and Psychiatry* 27: 161–86.

Han, Clara. 2012. *Life in Debt: Times of Care and Violence in Neoliberal Chile.* Berkeley: University of California Press.

———. 2013. "Suffering and Pictures of Anthropological Inquiry: A Response to Comments on *Life in Debt*." *Hau: Journal of Ethnographic Theory* 3 (1): 231–40.

Han, Hahrie. 2009. *Moved to Action: Motivation, Participation, and Inequality in American Politics.* Stanford, CA: Stanford University Press.

Harris, Gillian, Linda Connor, Andrew Bisits, and Nick Higginbotham. 2004. "'Seeing the Baby': Pleasures and Dilemmas of Ultrasound Technologies for Primiparous Australian Women." *Medical Anthropology Quarterly* 18 (1): 23–47.

Harvey, David. 2005. *A Brief History of Neoliberalism.* New York: Oxford University Press.

Hellinger, Daniel. 2011. "Defying the Iron Law of Oligarchy I: How Does 'El Pueblo' Conceive Democracy?" In *Venezuela's Bolivian Democracy: Participation,*

Politics, and Culture under Chávez, edited by David Smilde and Daniel Hellinger, 28–57. Durham, NC: Duke University Press.

————. 2016a. "Venezuela's Agony." Caracas Connect, June 2016. http://
democracyinamericas.org/caracas-connect-venezuelas-agony/. Accessed April 19,
2017.

————. 2016b. "Venezuela's Agony Intensifies." Caracas Connect, November 2016.
http://democracyinamericas.org/caracas-connect-november-2016-venezuelas-
agony-intensifies/. Accessed April 19, 2017.

Hellinger, Daniel, and Dorothea Melcher. 1988. "Venezuela: A Welfare State Out of
Gas?" Paper presented at Latin American Studies Association XXI International
Congress, Chicago, September 24–26.

Hetland, Gabriel. 2016. "How Severe Is Venezuela's Crisis?" *The Nation,* June 22.
https://www.thenation.com/article/how-severe-is-venezuelas-crisis/. Accessed
April 19, 2017.

————. 2017. "Why Is Venezuela Spriraling Out of Control?" *NACLA News,* April
28. http://nacla.org/news/2017/04/28/why-venezuela-spiraling-out-control.
Accessed April 30, 2017.

Hetland, Gabriel, and George Cicciarello-Maher. 2017. "The State of the Left in
Latin America: A Disillusioned Revolution in Venezuela." *North American Congress on Latin America and Jacobin Magazine,* June 2. http://nacla.org
/news/2017/10/04/state-left-latin-america-disillusioned-revolution-venezuela.
Accessed November 6, 2017.

High, Casey. 2009. "Remembering the Auca: Violence and Generational Memory in
Amazonian Ecuador." *Journal of the Royal Anthropological Institute* 15: 719–36.

Hopper, Kim. 2003. *Reckoning with Homelessness.* Ithaca, NY: Cornell University
Press.

Huenchuan, Sandra, ed. 2009. *Envejecimiento, derechos humanos y políticas públicas.*
Santiago, Chile: CEPAL.

El Informador. 2009. "INASS fortalece atención integral de adultos mayores en seis
estados del país." September 23. www.elinformador.com.ve/noticias/venezuela
/organismos/inass-fortalece-atencion-integral-adultos-mayores-seis-estados-
pais/4030. Accessed May 4, 2012.

Instituto Nacional de Estadística de Venezuela (INE). 2002. *XIII Censo General
(2001).* Caracas.

Izquierdo, Carolina. 2005. "When 'Health' Is Not Enough: Societal, Individual,
and Biomedical Assessments of Well-Being among the Matsigenka of the Peruvian Amazon." *Social Science and Medicine* 61: 767–83.

Jenkins, Janis, ed. 2011. *Pharmaceutical Self: The Global Shaping of Experience in an
Age of Psychopharmacology.* Santa Fe, NM: SAR Press.

Johnson, Avery. 2009. "Drug Firms See Poorer Nations as Sales Cure." *Wall Street
Journal,* July 7. http://online.wsj.com/article/SB124691259063602065.html.
Accessed June 13, 2011.

Johnston, Barbara Rose (Guest Ed.), Elizabeth Colson, Dean Falk, Graham St John,
John H. Bodley, Bonnie J. McCay, Alaka Wali, Carolyn Nordstrom, and Susan

Slyomovics. 2012. "On Happiness." Vital Topics Forum, *American Anthropologist* 114 (1): 6–18.

Kavedžija, Iza, and Harry Walker. 2015. "Happiness: Horizons of Purpose." Special Issue. *Hau: Journal of Ethnographic Theory* 5 (3).

Keane, Helen. 2008. "Pleasure and Discipline in the Uses of Ritalin." *International Journal of Drug Policy* 19 (5): 401–9.

Keane, Julian. 2016. "Venezuela Crisis: Caracas Hospital Shows Sorry State of Health System." BBS World Service, October 9. www.bbc.com/news/world-latin-america-37562058. Accessed April 19, 2017.

Kelly, Tobias. 2013. "A Life Less Miserable?" *Hau: Journal of Ethnographic Theory* 3 (1): 213–16.

Kirk, John. 2015. *Healthcare without Borders: Understanding Cuban Medical Internationalism.* Tallahassee: University Press of Florida.

Kirmayer, Laurence. 2004. "The Cultural Diversity of Healing: Meaning, Metaphor, and Mechanism." *British Medical Bulletin* 69: 33–48.

Kleinman, Arthur. 1997. "What Is Specific to Biomedicine?" In *Writing at the Margin: Discourse between Anthropology and Medicine,* 21–40. Berkeley: University of California Press.

Kohut, Meridith. 2017. "In Need of a Cure: Venezuelans Are Turning to Faith Healers as the Nation's Crisis Deepens." *National Geographic,* June 28. www.nationalgeographic.com/photography/proof/2017/06/venezuela-health-crisis-spirits-photography/. Accessed February 27, 2018.

Kozloff, Nikolas. 2005. "Hugo Chávez and the Politics of Race." *Venezuela Analysis,* October 15. https://venezuelanalysis.com/analysis/1414. Accessed November 8, 2016.

Kulick, Don. 2006. "Theory in Furs: Masochist Anthropology." *Current Anthropology* 47 (6): 933–52.

Lan, David. 1985. *Guns and Rain: Guerillas and Spirit Mediums in Zimbabwe.* Berkeley: University of California Press.

Lancaster, Roger. 1994. *Life Is Hard: Machismo, Danger, and the Intimacy of Power in Nicaragua.* Berkeley: University of California Press.

Lander, Edgardo. 2005. "Venezuelan Social Conflict in a Global Context." *Latin American Perspectives* 32 (2): 20–38.

Lander, Edgardo, and Luis Fierro. 1996. "The Impact of Neoliberal Adjustment in Venezuela, 1989–1993." *Latin American Perspectives* 23 (3): 50–73.

López Maya, Margarita. 2002. *Protesta y cultura en Venezuela: Los marcos de acción colectiva en 1999.* Buenos Aires: CLASCO.

López Maya, Margarita, David Smilde, and Keta Stephany. 2006. "Identades en movimiento (aspectos del marco de acción colectiva) de la protesta popular venezolana en 1999." *Espacio Abierto: Cuaderno Venezolano de Sociología* 15 (1–2): 197–219.

Low, Setha. 1988. "The Medicalization of Healing Cults in Latin America." *American Ethnologist* 15 (1): 136–54.

Luhrmann, Tanya. 2008. "'The Street Will Drive You Crazy': Why Homeless Psychotic Women in the Institutional Circuit in the United States Often Say No to Offers of Help." *American Journal of Psychiatry* 165 (1): 15–20.

———. 2009. "Uneasy Street." In *The Insecure American: How We Got Here and What We Should Do about It,* edited by Hugh Gusterson and Catherine Besterman, 207–33. Berkeley: University of California Press.

Marcano, Patricia. 2008. "Fármacos regresan a las boticas: De 9,800 medicamentos existentes sólo fallaron tres." *Últimas Noticias (Caracas),* March 1.

Margolies, Luise. 1984. "José Gregorio Hernández: The Historical Development of a Venezuelan Popular Saint." *Studies in Latin American Popular Culture* 3: 28–46.

María, Eva, Naomi Schiller, and Gregory Wilpert. 2017. "Debating the Bolivarian Revolution." *Jacobin,* May 19. www.jacobinmag.com/2017/05/debating-the-bolivarian-revolution. Accessed November 8, 2017.

Maribel Navas, Olga. 2008. "Vecinos se proponen rescatar espacios del Paseo Anauco." *Últimas Noticias (Caracas),* February 24, 8.

Martin, Emily. 2006. "The Pharmaceutical Person." *Biosocieties* 1: 273–87.

Martinez, Carlos, Michael Fox, and Jojo Farrell. 2010. *Venezuela Speaks! Voices from the Grassroots.* Oakland, CA: PM Press.

Martinez, Rebecca. 2005. "'What's Wrong with Me?' Cervical Cancer in Venezuela—Living in the Borderlands of Health, Disease, and Illness." *Social Science and Medicine* 61 (4): 797–808.

Maternowska, M. Catherine. 2006. *Reproducing Inequities: Poverty and the Politics of Population in Haiti.* New Brunswick, NJ: Rutgers University Press.

Mathews, Gordon, and Carolina Izquierdo, eds. 2009. *Pursuits of Happiness: Well-Being in Anthropological Perspective.* Oxford: Berghahn.

McCallum, Cecilia, and Ana Paula dos Reis. 2005. "Childbirth as Ritual in Brazil: Young Mothers' Experiences." *Ethnos* 70 (3): 335–60.

Mignone, Javier, Judith Bartlett, John O'Neil, and Treena Orchard. 2007. "Best Practices in Intercultural Health: Five Case Studies in Latin America." *Journal of Ethnobiology and Ethnomedicine* 3 (31): 1–11.

Ministerio de Salud y Desarrollo Social (MSDS). n.d. "¿Cómo conformar círculos de abuelos?" Caracas.

Mitchell, Lisa M. 2001. *Baby's First Picture: Ultrasound and the Politics of Fetal Subjects.* Toronto: University of Toronto Press.

Mitchell, Lisa M., and Eugenia Georges. 1997. "Cross-Cultural Cyborgs: Greek and Canadian Women's Discourses on Fetal Ultrasound." *Feminist Studies* 23 (2): 373–401.

Mol, Annemarie. 2008. *The Logic of Care: Health and the Problem of Patient Choice.* London: Routledge.

Morales, Nicolás, and W. Acosta Lastra. 1991. "The Grandparents Club: The Results of a Working Period." *Revista Cubana de Enfermería* 7 (1): 26–31.

Nading, Alex. 2012. "Dengue Mosquitos Are Single Mothers: Biopolitics Meets Ecological Aesthetics in Nicaraguan Community Health Work." *Cultural Anthropology* 27 (4): 572–96.

———. 2014. *Mosquito Trails: Ecology, Health, and the Politics of Entanglement.* Berkeley: University of California Press.

Naraindas, H., and C. Bastos. 2011. "Healing Holidays? Itinerant Patients, Therapeutic Locales, and the Quest for Health." *Medical Anthropology* 18: 1–6.

National Public Radio. 2007. "Santería Experiences Big League Surge." July 5. www.npr.org/templates/story/story.php?storyId = 11756310. Accessed August 16, 2011.

Nations, Marilyn, and Linda-Anne Rebhun. 1988. "Mystification of a Simple Solution: Oral Rehydration Therapy in Northeast Brazil." *Social Science and Medicine* 27 (1): 25–38.

Neuman, William. 2014. "As Catholic Church Seeks Proof, Venezuela Sees a Saint." *New York Times,* September 29. https://nyti.ms/1nBTIG0. Accessed April 18, 2017.

Nunley, Michael. 1988. "The Involvement of Families in Indian Psychiatry." *Culture, Medicine, and Psychiatry* 22: 317–53.

Ochoa, Marcia. 2014. *Queen for a Day: Transformistas, Beauty Queens, and the Performance of Femininity in Venezuela.* Durham, NC: Duke University Press.

O'Neil, John D. 1989. "The Cultural and Political Context of Patient Dissatisfaction in Cross-Cultural Clinical Encounters: A Canadian Inuit Study." *Medical Anthropology Quarterly* 3 (4): 325–44.

Organización Panaméricana de la Salud (OPS). 2006. *Barrio Adentro: Derecho a la salud e inclusión social en Venezuela.* Caracas: OPS / OMS para Venezuela.

Ortner, Sherry. 2016. "Dark Anthropology and Its Others: Theory since the Eighties." *Hau: Journal of Ethnographic Theory* 6 (1): 47–73.

Paley, Julia. 2001. *Marketing Democracy: Power and Social Movements in Post-Dictatorship Chile.* Berkeley: University of California Press.

Palmer, Steven. 2003. *From Popular Medicine to Medical Populism: Doctors, Healers, and Public Power in Costa Rica, 1800–1940.* Durham, NC: Duke University Press.

Pan American Health Organization (PAHO). 2012. *Health in the Americas: 2012 Edition.* Washington, DC: PAHO.

Paullier, Juan. 2011. "Venezuela, espiritismo y santería." BBC Mundo, October 18. www.bbc.com/mundo/noticias/2011/10/111017_venezuela_religion_santeria_espiritismo_jp.shtml. Accessed January 20, 2017.

PBS NewsHour. 2017. "Venezuela's Hospitals Face Crisis as Meds Run Low." March 26. www.pbs.org/newshour/show/venezuela-hospitals-face-crisis-meds-run-low.

Perez, Christina. 2008. *Caring for Them from Birth to Death: The Practice of Community-Based Cuban Medicine.* Lanham, MD: Rowman and Littlefield.

Pestano, Andrew. 2016. "Venezuelan President to Expand Welfare Health Reform amid Economic Crisis." UPI, August 22. www.upi.com/Top_News/World-News/2016/08/22/Venezuelan-president-to-expand-welfare-health-program-amid-economic-crisis/8431471872437/. Accessed April 19, 2017.

———. 2017. "Venezuela: 75% of Population Lost 19 Pounds amid Crisis." UPI, February 19. www.upi.com/Venezuela-75-of-population-lost-19-pounds-amid-crisis/2441487523377/. Accessed November 15, 2017.

Petersen, Margit Anne, Lotte Stig Nørgaard, and Janine Marie Traulsen. 2015. "Pursuing Pleasures of Productivity: University Students' Use of Prescription Stimulants for Enhancement and the Moral Uncertainty of Making Work Fun." *Culture, Medicine, and Psychiatry* 39 (4): 665–79.

Pettigrew, Judith. 2013. *Maoists at the Hearth: Everyday Life in Nepal's Civil War.* Philadelphia: University of Pennsylvania Press.

Pollak-Eltz, Angelina. 1982. *Folk-Medicine in Venezuela.* Acta Ethnologica et Linguistica No. 53. Vienna: Elgelbert Stiglmayr.

Prentice, Rachel. 2012. *Bodies in Formation: An Ethnography of Anatomy and Surgery Education.* Durham, NC: Duke University Press.

Programa Venezolano de Educación-Acción en Derechos Humanos (PROVEA). 2007. "Situación de los derechos humanos en Venezuela: Informe anual octubre /septiembre." Caracas: PROVEA. www.derechos.org.ve/informes-anuales /informe-anual-2007/. Accessed February 22, 2015.

———. 2011. "MPPCI: Un millón 926.503 pensionados en Venezuela." December 19. www.derechos.org.ve/2011/12/19.

Race, Kane. 2009. *Pleasure Consuming Medicine: The Queer Politics of Drugs.* Durham, NC: Duke University Press.

———. 2017. "Thinking with Pleasure: Experimenting with Drugs and Drug Research." *International Journal of Drug Policy* 49: 144–49.

Reardon, Juan. 2011. "Venezuela Marks Five Years of Mission Negra Hipolita." *Venezuela Analysis,* January 14. https://venezuelanalysis.com/news/5936. Accessed February 7, 2017.

Reporte (Reporte de la Economía). 2008. "Debatirán inclusión de medicina tradicional en Ley de Salud." July 21. www.guia.com.ve/noti/26127/debatiran-inclusion-de-medicina-tradional-en-ley-de-salud. Accessed February 23, 2012.

Robbins, Joel. 2013. "Beyond the Suffering Subject: Toward an Anthropology of the Good." *Journal of the Royal Anthropological Institute* 19: 447–62.

Roberts, Elizabeth. 2012a. *God's Laboratory: Assisted Reproduction in the Andes.* Berkeley: University of California Press.

———. 2012b. "Scars of Nation: Surgical Penetration and the Ecuadorian State." *Journal of Latin American and Caribbean Anthropology* 17 (2): 215–37.

Salter, Lee, and Dave Weltman. 2011. "Class, Nationalism, and News: The BBC's Reporting of Hugo Chávez and the Bolivarian Revolution." *International Journal of Media and Cultural Politics* 7 (3): 253–73.

Samet, Robert, and Naomi Schiller. 2017. "All Populisms are not Created Equal." *Anthropology News* 58 (3): e63–e70.

Sarmiendo Garmendia, Mabel. 2008. "Indigentes hacen de las suya." *Últimas Noticias (Caracas),* May 23, 3.

Scheper-Hughes, Nancy. 1993. *Death without Weeping: The Violence of Everyday Life in Brazil.* Berkeley: University of California Press.

Scheper-Hughes, Nancy, and Margaret Lock. 1987. "The Mindful Body: A Prolegomenon to Future Work in Medical Anthropology." *Medical Anthropology Quarterly* 1 (1): 6–41.

Schielke, Samuli. 2015. *Egypt in the Future Tense: Hope, Frustration, and Ambivalence before and after 2011.* Bloomington: Indiana University Press.

Schiller, Naomi. 2013. "Reckoning with Press Freedom: Community Media, Liberalism, and the Processual State in Caracas, Venezuela." *American Ethnologist* 40 (3): 540–54.

———. 2018. *Channeling the State: Community Media and Popular Politics in Venezuela.* Durham, NC: Duke University Press.

Scott, James. 1976. *The Moral Economy of the Peasant: Subsistence and Rebellion in Southeast Asia.* New Haven, CT: Yale University Press.

Sen, Amartya. 2002. "Health: Perception versus Observation." *British Medical Journal* 324: 860–61.

Shah, Alpa. 2014. "'The Muck of the Past': Revolution, Social Transformation, and the Maoists in India." *Journal of the Royal Anthropological Institute* 20: 337–56.

Smilde, David. 2008. "The Social Structure of Hugo Chávez." *Contexts* 7: 38–43.

———. 2016. "Chavismo Full Circle." *New York Times,* October 31. www.nytimes.com/2016/11/01/opinion/chavismo-full-circle.html?_r=1. Accessed April 19, 2017.

Smilde, David, and Daniel Hellinger. 2011. *Venezuela's Bolivarian Democracy: Participation, Politics, and Culture under Chávez.* Durham, NC: Duke University Press.

Smith-Oka, Vania. 2012. "Bodies of Risk: Constructing Motherhood in a Mexican Public Hospital." *Social Science and Medicine* 75 (12): 2275–82.

———. 2013. "Managing Labor and Delivery among Impoverished Populations in Mexico: Cervical Examinations as Bureaucratic Practice." *American Anthropologist* 115 (4): 595–607.

Solomon, Harris. 2011. "Affective Journeys: The Emotional Structuring of Medical Tourism in India." *Anthropology and Medicine* 18 (1): 105–18.

Sowell, David. 2001. *The Tale of Healer Miguel Perdomo Neira: Medicine, Ideologies and Power in the Nineteenth-century Andes.* Wilmington, DE: Scholarly Resources.

Starr, Paul. 1982. *The Social Transformation of American Medicine.* New York: Basic Books.

Stefanoni, Pablo. 2017. "¿Por qué no bajan de los cerros? Entrevista a Alejandro Velasco." *Nueva Sociedad,* June. http://nuso.org/articulo/venezuela-por-que-no-bajan-de-los-cerros/. Accessed November 8, 2017.

Taussig, Michael. 1980. "Reification and the Consciousness of the Patient." *Social Science and Medicine* 14 (1): 3–13.

———. 1997. *The Magic of the State.* New York: Routledge.

Telesur TV. 2016. "5,000 New Doctors Graduate in Venezuela." October 9. www.telesurtv.net/english/news/5000-New-Doctors-Graduate-in-Venezuela-20161009–0003.html. Accessed April 19, 2017.

Thomassen, Bjørn. 2012. "Notes towards an Anthropology of Political Revolutions." *Comparative Studies in Society and History* 54 (3): 679–706.

Tinker Salas, Miguel. 2009. *The Enduring Legacy: Oil, Culture, and Society in Venezuela.* Durham, NC: Duke University Press.

———. 2015. *Venezuela: What Everyone Needs to Know.* Oxford: Oxford University Press.

Trnka, Susanna. 2017. "Efficacious Holidays: The Therapeutic Dimensions of Pleasure and Discipline in Czech Respiratory Spas." *Medical Anthropology Quarterly* 32 (1): 42–58.

Tuck, Eve. 2009. "Suspending Damage: A Letter to Communities." *Harvard Educational Review* 79 (3): 409–27.

United Nations Children's Fund (UNICEF). 2014. *The State of the World's Children 2015: Reimagine the Future.* New York: UNICEF.

United Nations Development Programme (UNDP). 2010. *Human Development Report 2010.* New York: UNDP.

———. 2015. *Human Development Report 2015: Work for Human Development.* New York: UNDP.

U.S. Department of State. n.d. "U.S. Embassy Movement Policy." Venezuela: Safety and Security. https://travel.state.gov/content/passports/en/country/venezuela .html. Accessed December 5, 2016.

Valencia, Cristobal. 2015. *We Are the State! Barrio Activism in Venezuela's Bolivarian Revolution.* Tucson: University of Arizona Press.

Van Dongen, Els, and Riekje Elema. 2001. "The Art of Touching: The Culture of 'Body Work' in Nursing." *Anthropology and Medicine* 8 (2–3): 149–62.

Vega, Rosalynn. 2018. "How Natural Birth Became Inaccessible to the Poor." *Sapiens,* April 6. www.sapiens.org/body/indigenous-midwives-mexico/. Accessed April 10, 2018.

Velasco, Alejandro. 2015. *Barrio Rising: Urban Popular Politics and the Making of Modern Venezuela.* Berkeley: University of California Press.

Venezuela Analysis. 2006. "Venezuela Launches Social Mission Aimed at Helping the Most Vulnerable." *Venezuela Analysis,* January 16. https://venezuelanalysis .com/news/1570. Accessed April 19, 2017.

Villasana López, Pedro Enrique. 2010. "De Alma Ata a Barrio Adentro: Una aproximación al sentido histórico de las metamorfosis del discurso de la participación en salud en Venezuela." In *De la participación en salud a la construcción del poder popular,* edited by Johanna Lévy and Miguel Malo, 31–67. Maracay, Venezuela: Instituto de Altos Estudios Dr. Arnoldo Gabaldón.

Waitzkin, Howard. 1991. *The Politics of Medical Encounters: How Patients and Doctors Deal with Social Problems.* New Haven, CT: Yale University Press.

Waitzkin, Howard, Celia Iriart, Alfredo Estrada, and Silvia Lamadrid. 2001. "Social Medicine Then and Now: Lessons from Latin America." *American Journal of Public Health* 91 (10): 1592–1601.

Weddle, Cody. 2016. "Mission Fights Homelessness and Addiction on Venezuela Streets." Telesur TV, September 26. www.telesurtv.net/english/news/Mission-

Fights-Homelessness-and-Addiction-on-Venezuela-Streets-20160926–0015
.html. Accessed February 7, 2017.

Weisbrot, Mark, Rebecca Ray, and Luis Sandoval. 2009. *The Chávez Administration at 10 Years: The Economy and Social Indicators*. Washington, DC: Center for Economic and Policy Research.

Wendland, Claire. 2010. *A Heart for the Work: Journeys through an African Medical School*. Chicago: University of Chicago Press.

West, Candace. 1984. "Turn-Taking in Doctor-Patient Dialogues." In *Routine Complications: Troubles with Talk between Doctors and Patients*, edited by Candace West, 51–70. Bloomington: Indiana University Press.

Westhoff, W.W., R. Rodriguez, C. Cousins, and R.J. McDermott. 2010. "Cuban Healthcare Providers in Venezuela: A Case Study." *Public Health* 124: 519–24.

Whiteford, Linda, and Laurence Branch. 2008. *Primary Health Care in Cuba: The Other Revolution*. New York: Rowman and Littlefield.

Whitmarsh, Ian, and Elizabeth Roberts, eds. 2015. "Nonsecular Medical Anthropology." Special Issue. *Medical Anthropology: Cross-Cultural Studies in Health and Illness* 35 (3).

Wilpert, Gregory. 2007. *Changing Venezuela by Taking Power: The History and Politics of the Chávez Government*. London: Verso.

———. 2011. "An Assessment of Venezuela's Bolivarian Revolution at Twelve Years." *Venezuela Analysis,* http://venezuelanalysis.com/analysis/5971. Accessed July 2, 2011.

Wolf, Eric. 1969. *Peasant Wars of the Twentieth Century*. New York: Harper & Row.

World Health Organization (WHO). 2001. *Legal Status of Traditional Medicine and Complementary/Alternative Medicine: A Worldwide Review*. http://apps.who.int/medicinedocs/en/d/Jh2943e/1.html. Accessed June 13, 2011.

Yates-Doerr, Emily. 2012. "The Weight of the Self: Care and Compassion in Guatemalan Dietary Choices." *Medical Anthropology Quarterly* 26 (1): 136–58.

Žižek, Slavoj. 1993. "Enjoy Your Nation as Yourself!" In *Tarrying with the Negative: Kant, Hegel, and the Critique of Ideology*. Durham, NC: Duke University Press.

Zulawski, Ann. 2007. *Unequal Cures: Public Health and Political Change in Bolivia, 1900–1950*. Durham, NC: Duke University Press.

INDEX

NOTE: Page numbers in *italics* denote illustrations.

acupuncture, 72, 73, 86, 94

Adelson, Naomi, 163n69

Afro-Cuban religion. *See* santería

Afro-Venezuelans: racist attacks on
Chávez's heritage, 18. *See also* Bolívar,
Hipólita; empowerment of historically
disenfranchised groups; espiritismo
(cult of María Lionza); marginalization
of historically disenfranchised groups

aging population. *See* Grandparents Clubs
(Clubes de Abuelos); older adults

Allende, Salvador, 166n8

alternative medicine: as term, 165n1. *See
also* popular medicine

Andaya, Elise, 168n40

aprovechando (making the most of government services): community health
workers and pressure for, 79–80; Cuban
doctor complaints about patient lack of,
82; definition of, 79; indigente nonparticipation in, and displeasure of community volunteers, 135, 140–43; as
moral obligation/imperative, 135, 140–
41; participación distinguished from,
122; patient nonparticipation in, 82,
96–97; and pleasure of access in light
of historical hunger for health care,
80–81, 122; and specialized care as
limited, 81–82; as transformative,
140

Argentina, Grandparents Clubs in, 169n6

Asian-derived health practices, popularity
of, 86

asthma, 38, 39, 82

ayahuasca ceremonies, 8

Baer, Hans, 166n5

bailoterapia (dance therapy), 2–3, *2*, 51, 73,
104, 109

Barrio Adentro (Inside the Barrio): overview, 1, 17, 19–21; affordability of,
75–76, 87–88, 95; controversies sur-
rounding, 21; as corruption free, patient
view of, 74; Cuban biopsychosocial
model of medicine and, 20, 57–59;
Cuban Family Doctor program and, 20,
96; Cuba-Venezuela agreement and,
19–20, 36, 66, 162n54; doctor-to-patient
ratio in, 22; establishment of, 20, 35;
freedom of choice in, 76, 79, 85, 95–97;
funding of, via oil wealth, 17; hospital
system rehabilitation (Barrio Adentro
III), 20; improved access to health care
and, 22–24, 163nn65,69; mandated
compliance not part of Chávez-era
model, 82, 96–97; meaning of the term,
45, 140; *medicina integral* (integrated/
comprehensive medicine) approach,
57–60; numbers of clinics opened, 22,
35, 95; patient charts not maintained in
(except for infant immunizations), 96,
166n10, 168n41; post-Chávez era and

Barrio Adentro *(continued)*
difficulties of, 150–53; publicity for,
59–60; public support for, 20–21; specialized health center (Barrio Adentro
II, CDI and SRI), 20, 151, 152; three
levels of care of, 20; Venezuelan doctors,
difficulty of recruiting to, 20, 44; violent attacks on clinics and hospitals, 21,
151. *See also aprovechando* (making the
most of government services); community-based medicine (Barrio Adentro I
clinics); community health workers of
Barrio Adentro; Cuba; doctors; empowerment of historically disenfranchised
groups; *participación popular* (popular
participation); specialized care
Barrio Adentro Rehabilitation Centers. *See*
SRI
barrios: definition of, 140, 159n1; history of,
126; post-Chávez government protests
in, 150; resignification of, as capable of
promoting health, 11–12, 43, 44–46; as
typical research site in urban Venezuela,
27. *See also* community-based medicine
(Barrio Adentro I clinics); homelessness
and the homeless
BBC News, 29. *See also* media coverage
beauty norms, 50
Béhague, Dominique, 160n10
belonging. *See* national belonging
Bernstein, Alyssa, 59, 160n11
biomedicalized subject, 77, 85
biomedicine: biopsychosocial model/
integrated medicine, 20, 57–59; caution
in using, patient worldview of, 72–75,
77–78, 79; definition of, 5, 159n4;
income inequalities and historical lack
of access to, 5–6, 11; licensing and, 70,
166n6; mandated compliance enforced
in Cuban model of, 96, 97, 168n40;
mandated compliance not part of
Chávez-era model of, 82, 96–97; medical gaze and, 58; medical profiling, 6; as
"monotheistic" and seeking to delegitimize popular medical traditions, 70–71,
97, 166nn5–6,8; and religion, intertwin-
ing of, 31–35, 85–87, 164n1; universal
access guaranteed in 1999 Constitution,

17, *18*, 20–21, 92–93; universal access to,
as promise of Bolivarian Revolution,
5–6; and the white coat, 62, 166n6. *See
also* Barrio Adentro; drugs; marginalization of historically disenfranchised
groups; medical pluralism; popular
medicine; private health care
biophysical health. *See under* health
Blumhagen, Dan, 166n6
Bolívar, Hipólita, 129–30
Bolivarian Revolution: inevitable incompleteness of, 142; as term, 17. *See also*
Chávez-era government
Bolívar, Simón (el Libertador), 17, 26,
129–30
Bolivia: Cuban medical internationalism
and, 59, 160n11; and pleasurable dimensions of public health care, 160n11;
popular medical traditions recognized
in, 95
Brazil, public health care, 54, 159–60nn6–7
Briggs, Charles, 6
Brotherton, Sean, 97

capitalism. *See* economics; neoliberalism
Caracas: Cuban medical relief after natural
disaster in, 20; historic district of, 25;
municipalities of, mentioned, 16,
163n78. *See also* barrios; Libertador
municipality; methodology; Santa
Teresa (residential district); spatial
segregation; Venezuela
Caracazo (1989 protest against neoliberal
austerity), 16, 17
Castro, Raul, 72
Catholicism: canonization of José Gregorio
Hernández, 33, 164n6; and conviction
that health care should be available to
all, 20; percentage of population in, 85;
and spiritual healing traditions, 85
Catia barrio, 36–37, *37*
CDI (Centros de Diagnóstico Integral,
Comprehensive Diagnostic Centers—
Barrio Adentro II), 20, 151, 152
Centers of Social Inclusion, 138
Chacao Municipality, 16
Chávez-era government: Cuban presence in
Venezuela, 65–66; legacy of, 156–57;

love and compassion as basis of publicity for, 59–60; as "twenty-first-century socialism," 18; "Venezuela: Ahora es de todos" (Now Venezuela belongs to everyone), 17, 121. *See also* Chávez-era government programs; Chávez, Hugo; citizenship; Constitution of Venezuela (1999); media coverage; national belonging; oil wealth; right-wing opposition to Chávez-era government

Chávez-era government programs: education missions (e.g. Misión Ribas), 18–19, 23, 50, 170n15; improvements in population health, 23–24; oil wealth as funding, 17, 19, 162n52; social missions, 18–19; soup kitchens (*casas de alimentación*), 23, 124, 136; for specialized treatment needs, 76–77, 82; subsidized grocery stores (Misión Mercal), 23; trade and aid programs with Latin America and the Caribbean, 18. *See also aprovechando* (making the most of government services); Barrio Adentro (Inside the Barrio); empowerment of historically disenfranchised groups; Grandparents Clubs (Clubes de Abuelos); Negra Hipólita mission (homeless outreach program); *participación popular* (popular participation); pleasures of Venezuelan government health care

Chávez, Hugo: Afro-Venezuelan and indigenous heritage of, 18; *Aló Presidente* (television show), 129; approval ratings of, 17; death of, 21, 148; electoral campaigns of, 5, 17, 18, 139; failed coup attempt against (2002), 18, 72; failed coup attempt by (1992), 17; length of presidency, 21; personal interventions by, 78; on popular medicine, 95; publicity photos of, emphasizing love and compassion, 60; racist attacks on, 18; recall referendum against (2004), 18; and social justice, emphasis on, 5–6, 18–19; "We Want to End Poverty? Let's Give Power to the Poor," 170n15

childbirth: prenatal care, 82, 168n40; in public hospitals, 159–60nn5–6,10,

161n25; and violent attacks on health care centers, 151

children's health, post-Chávez era and declines in, 150–51, 152–53. *See also* infant mortality rates

Chile, community health activism in, 168–69n1

China, health promotion practices of ("life cultivation arts"), 8

Chinese traditional medicine, 8, 91–92; acupuncture, 72, 73, 86, 94

citizenship: classical liberal idea of, 161n27; and demarginalization, 140, 141–43, 171n17; reciprocity and, 156–57; Venezuelan, as member of corporate national body, 161n27; Venezuelan, framed as shared ownership of oil wealth, 12, 13–14, 145, 146. *See also* democratic government; national belonging

class: and expectation of humanitarianism/compassion/solidarity from doctors, 146, 171n2; and right-wing opposition to Chávez/Maduro governance, 149–50; and spatial segregation, 44. *See also* empowerment of historically disenfranchised groups; income inequality; marginalization of historically disenfranchised groups; social inequalities; structural inequalities

clinics of Barrio Adentro. *See* community-based medicine (Barrio Adentro I clinics)

Clubes de Abuelos. *See* Grandparents Clubs

Colombia, health care, 75–76

Comité de Salud. *See* Health Committees

community-based medicine (Barrio Adentro I clinics): overview, 20, 31, 35–36; access to and need for, 42–44; architecture of clinics, 45, *50*, 147; doctor-saint José Gregorio as symbolic of, 35, 36, 59; empowerment of marginalized groups via, 41, 43, 95, 171n16; house calls, 38, 48, 51; and inclusion of the excluded (*los excluidos*), 42–44; legacy of right to, 157; limitations of, 41–42; locations of clinics, 35–37, 45, *65*, 102; pre-Chávez

and members, 105; and participation as transformative practice, 121, 122–23; and personal transformation, 108–12, 121, 122–23, 169nn11–12,18; pleasures of, 3, 11, 103–4, 105; in post-Chávez era, 150; and public spaces, repurposing of, 45, 116–20, *117, 119–20*; socializing and psychological well-being as promoted by, 105, 109; women as primary participants in, 104, 168–69n1

grocery stores, government subsidized (Misión Mercal), 23

Guatemala: and pleasure in medicine, 8; and public health programs, 160n11

Guevara, Ché, 166n8

Haiti, public health treatment of the poor, 160n10

Han, Hahrie, 169n10

happiness, as term, 10, 161n23

health: decline of, in post-Chávez era, 150–55; definitions and assessments of, by medical professionals vs. patients, 23, 24, 163n69. *See also* Chávez-era government programs; health promotion; infant mortality rates; life expectancy

—BIOPHYSICAL HEALTH: health policy, and cultural context of medical interventions, 153–54; material improvements to, as pleasure, 10, 108–9; reductionistic analyses of, 13

Health Committees (Comité de Salud), 28–29, 101–2. *See also* community health workers

health policy, and cultural context of medical interventions, 153–54

health promotion: Chinese "life cultivation arts," 8; expansion of health education, 93; *jornadas de salud* (health fairs), 45; natural and traditional foods, 94; repurposing public spaces for, 45. *See also* community health workers of Barrio Adentro; Grandparents Clubs (Clubes de Abuelos); Negra Hipólita mission (homeless outreach program)

Hernández, José Gregorio (doctor-saint), *32*; overview, 31–32; as biomedical "doctor of the poor" (*el médico de los pobres*), 32–33, 34–35, 59; Catholic Church and canonization of, 33, 164n6; community-based medicine as inspired by, 35, 36, 59; death of, 33; humanitarianism/compassion/solidarity of doctors as symbolized by, 34–35, 44, 59; mystical healing powers, cult of, 33–34, 86, 87, 88, 90, 91, 167nn27,29

historically marginalized/disenfranchised groups: definition of, 11. *See also* empowerment of historically disenfranchised groups; marginalization of historically disenfranchised groups

homelessness and the homeless (*personas sin techo*): and constitutional housing guarantees, 126; and incomplete rehabilitation, 135; indigentes defined as the most vulnerable and marginalized among, 126–27; numbers of, 126–27; squatters, 124–25, 126; structural forces and intractability of, 124, 126. *See also* Negra Hipólita mission (homeless outreach program)

homeopathy, 48, 73, 86, 94

housing: for doctors, 102; universal access guaranteed in 1999 Constitution, 17, 126. *See also* homelessness

humanitarianism: as challenged by indigente (homeless) patients, 138–39; Chávez on the Negra Hipólita homeless mission, 129; *humanitario* (humanitarian) vs. *materialista/mercantilista* (materialist) practices of doctors, 53–54, 57–58, 61–64, 66. *See also* compassion; doctors—humanitarianism/compassion/solidarity expected of good doctors

hypertension, 38, 52, 82, 151

income inequality: Chávez era and improvements in, 24, 91; and historical access/lack of access to biomedicine, 5–6, 11; poverty rates as increasing under neoliberalism, 16, 162n39; pre-Chávez neoliberal austerity measures and worsening of, 161; worst levels in Latin America, in Venezuela, 14. *See also* inequalities; neoliberalism

dominance and, 70–71, 97, 166nn5–6,8; the medical gaze and, 58; medical profiling and, 6; in public health services, generally, 6–7, 54, 66–67, 159–60nn5–6,10–11, 165n21; socialist governments and, 71, 97; specific physician behaviors and, 6–7, 54, 56–57, 159n5, 160n10; status asymmetries and, 54, 56–57, 159–60n6. *See also* empowerment of historically disenfranchised groups; *marginalidad* (marginality, social exclusion)

Martinez, Rebecca, 6

materialista/mercantilista (materialist) vs. *humanitario* (humanitarian) practices of doctors, 53–54, 57–58, 61–64, 66

Maternowska, Catherine, 160n10

Matsigenka people, 23

Maya people, 165n21

media coverage, of post-Chávez era, 148, 152

—OF CHÁVEZ ERA: comparisons of Trump and Chávez in, 29; ethnography as corrective to, 29; historically privileged groups as favored in, 29; on indigentes, 127–28; negative framing of Barrio Adentro, 21; negative framing of Bolivarian Venezuela, 28, 40, 164n8; racist attacks on Chávez in, 17–18; on *santería,* 90, 167n26; statistics on bias in, 29

medical anthropology: focus on negative aspects of health care in, 7–8, 160–61n14; nonsecular, 164n1; and pleasure as explicit focus of analysis, 8–9, 160n11, 161n23. *See also* ethnography; methodology; pleasure in medicine

medical internationalism. *See* Cuba—medical internationalism of

medical pluralism: overview, 5, 69–70; acupuncture and, 72, 73, 86, 94; biomedical hegemony/delegitimization of popular medicine, 70–71, 97, 166nn5–6,8; Chávez government support for, 69–70, 71, 92–98; definition of, 69; and empowerment, 70, 71, 92–98; and freedom of choice, 76, 79, 85, 95–97; historical practices, 88; homeopathy and, 48, 73, 86, 94; medical worldview

of participants, 78–79; participant narratives of, 71–78; selective use of biomedicine in, 75, 79, 86–88, 92, 94–95; separation of healing systems as separate entities for sake of discussion, 165n2. *See also* biomedicine; popular medicine

medical profiling, definition of, 6

medicine. *See* biomedicine; medical pluralism; popular medicine

meditation, 86

methodology: as corrective to media misrepresentation, 29; field site, 24–27, *25–26,* 163n78; and government interference, lack of, 29, 163–64n85; research methods, 27–29, 83, 163–64nn82,83,85, 166n15; and trust, 28–29, 163–64n85

Mexico, and childbirth of low-income indigenous women, 159n5

military, health care involvement, 14, 40, 48, 62, 75, 87

Ministry for Popular Participation and Social Development (MINPADES), 130

Ministry of Education, 14

Ministry of Health (MSAS), 14

Miraflores, 76–77, 163nn78,81,82

Misión Barrio Adentro. *See* Barrio Adentro

Misión Negra Hipólita. *See* Negra Hipólita mission (homeless outreach program)

Nading, Alex, 160n11

national belonging: Chávez-era health care and sense of, 12, 144–45; community-based biomedicine and sense of, 46, 47; doctor-patient interactions and sense of, 54–55, 56–57, 64, 165n21; pleasure of, 142–43. *See also* citizenship; democratic government

National Commission of Complementary Therapies (CONATEC), 94

National Institute of Geriatrics, 94, 111

Nations, Marilyn, 54

naturopathic medicine, 78, 94

Negra Hipólita mission (homeless outreach program): citizenship as linked with rehabilitation, 140, 171n17; complaints and shut-down of facilities, 135–37; distant rehabilitation institutions,

participación popular (popular participation): *aprovechando* distinguished from, 122; and constitutional change to participatory democracy, 120, 170n20; definition of, 121; as motivation, 105–6; nonparticipation as source of displeasure, 139–43, 145, 171n17; and oil wealth distribution discourse, 121; pleasure of, 122–23; as state official discourse, 120–21, 139–43, 145, 170–71nn15–17; as transformative practice, 121–23, 140

participatory democracy, Venezuela as, 120, 149, 156–57, 170n20. *See also* citizenship; democratic government

PDVSA (national oil company), 17, 19, 77. *See also* oil wealth

Pentecostalism, 85

people of color. *See* Afro-Venezuelans; empowerment of historically disenfranchised groups; indigenous people; marginalization of historically disenfranchised groups

Perez, Christina, 57–58, 96, 168n40

personas sin techo. *See* homelessness and the homeless

Peru, and indigenous health, 23

pharmaceuticals. *See* drugs

physical therapy, 4, 51, 73, 94

Plaza Bolívar, 118

pleasure: of community volunteers in homeless rehabilitation program, 124, 130–31, 133; as guiding ethic of revolutions, 156; national identity as form of, 142–43; as term, 10, 161n23. *See also* displeasure

pleasure in medicine: as explicit focus of anthropological analysis, 8–9, 160n11, 161n23; health policy and cultural contexts of, 153–54; moral injunction against drugs and, 8; and popular medical care for health and wellness, 91–92; as "surplus effects" of treatment, 9

pleasures of Venezuelan government health care: overview, 3–5, 30, 144–47; of access, in light of historical hunger for health care, 80–81, 122; and biophysical health, material improvements to, 10; and biophysical health, reductionistic

analyses as challenged by, 13; of community health workers in Barrio Adentro, 11, 12, 103, 105, 114–16; compared to experience in United States, 61; in dentistry, 60–61; and doctor-patient encounters, 10–11, 67; empowerment as, generally, 11–13; as expression of approval of the Chávez government, 12; freedom of choice in Barrio Adentro, 76, 79, 95–97; of Grandparents Clubs, 3, 11, 103–4, 105; of heeding the call to participation, 12; of increasing social equality, 11; and national belonging/citizenship, 12; *participación* and, 122–23; pleasure as term, 10, 161n23; and popular medicine, state respect for, 71; and post-Chávez era, 152; as resignifying marginalized neighborhoods, 11–12, 43, 44–46, 119–20; as sensual and social pleasures, 10–11

poder popular (popular power), 120–21

political empowerment. *See* empowerment of historically disenfranchised groups

Pollak-Eltz, Angelina, 88, 167n20

poor and working-class people. *See* barrios; empowerment of historically disenfranchised groups; homelessness; inequalities; marginalization of historically disenfranchised groups; neoliberalism

popular medicine: acupuncture, 72, 73, 86, 94; biomedicine as seeking to delegitimize, 70–71, 97, 166nn5–6,8; and biomedicine, permeable boundaries with, 86–87, 92; Chávez-era government recognition of and respect for, 69–70, 71, 85, 92, 93–95, 96–98, 168n38; commitment to, 3, 92; community health workers with preference for, 77–78; constitutional and legislative protections for, 94, 95; definition of, 69, 165n1; economic and political unrest as theory of popularity of, 91, 167–68nn29,31; empirical medicine, 85–86; health and wellness as goal of, 91–92; and historically marginalized groups, 85, 166n18; homeopathy, 48, 73, 86, 94; home remedies, 73, 78, 86, 87; increased usage of, in addition to biomedicine

popular medicine *(continued)*
access, 85, 88–90, 91; lack of biomedicine as theory of popularity of, 91, 167n27; medicine shops and suppliers (spiritual and plant-based healing), 69, 89–90, *89*, 167n25; mystical hospitals, 86–87; natural medicines set in opposition to pharmaceuticals, 84; naturopathic medicine, 78, 94; negative stereotypes of, 71; pleasure of government respect for, 71; spiritual healing traditions, 85–87, 91, 167nn19–20,25–27,29. *See also* biomedicine; medical pluralism
popular participation. *See participación popular* (popular participation)
popular power (*poder popular*), 120–21, 139
Portugal, Grandparents Clubs in, 169n6
post-Chávez Venezuela: overview, 21–22, 147–53; and deterioration of Chávez era programs, 21–22, 147, 150, 151–53; disillusionment and, 149–50; economic crisis of, 21–22, 148–49; food insecurity and malnutrition, 148–49, 150; health care, shortages and difficulties of, 150–53; health, decline in, 150–55; and legacy of Chávez era, 156–57; media coverage of, 148, 152; political instability of, 147–48, 149–50, 172n6; and violent attacks on Barrio Adentro clinics and hospitals, 21, 151; violent right-wing opposition to, 148, 149–50, 151
poverty rates, neoliberal austerity and increase in, 16, 162n39
pre-Chávez Venezuela: democratic rule in, continuous, 14; economic crises of 1980s and 1990s, 15; economic interventions to promote social welfare, 14; failed coup attempt (1992), 17; Fourth Republic, 51; with highest per capita debt in Latin America, 15; with highest per capita income in Latin America, 14; lack of programs for older adults, 3; neoliberal austerity measures in, 15–17; and oil prices, falling of, 15; oil-wealth redistribution projects of, 14; and oil wealth redistribution, promises for, 12, 13–14; social welfare system, 14; "Ven-

ezuelan exceptionalism" of, 14. *See also* Chávez-era government
—PUBLIC HEALTH CARE: compared with Barrio Adentro community-based health care, overview of, 37–41; doctor-patient interactions, 54, 56; doctors' absence from the barrio, 42–44; expansion of, 14; as fragmented, 14–15, 27, 77; long-term doctor-patient relationships established in, 164–65n2; neoliberal austerity practices, 16; as reinforcing the marginalization of vulnerable groups, 6–7
private health care: allegations of diversions of equipment and supplies to, from public facilities, 41, 74, 150; allegations of payoffs to doctors from prescriptions, 74; Ecuador and pleasure in, 67; humanitarianism/compassion/solidarity as missing in, 53, 54; malpractice by, 75; patient preference for Barrio Adentro despite having the resources for, 72–75, 79; petitions for specialized care in, 76–77, 82; pharmaceutical mismanagement and, 73–74; in post-Chávez Venezuela, 151; in pre-Chávez Venezuela, 22; preference for, and right-wing opposition to Barrio Adentro, 40–41
public health care: community health workers, history of, 170n21; general experience of, as reinforcing the marginalization of vulnerable groups, 6–7, 54, 66–67, 159–60nn5–6,10–11, 165n21; mandated compliance enforced in Cuban model of, 96, 97, 168n40; mandated compliance not part of Chávez model-era of, 82, 96–97; post-Chávez shortages and difficulties of, 150–55; United States and stigma of, 146, 171n3. *See also* Barrio Adentro (Inside the Barrio); Chávez-era government programs; pre-Chávez Venezuela—public health care
public spaces: Barrio Adentro and repurposing of, 45; Grandparents Clubs and repurposing of, 45, 116–20, *117*, *119–20*; and indigentes, removal from, 128–29, 135–36, 137; urban recuperation of, 128–29, 140

quality of life. *See* health; standard of living

race and ethnicity: racist attacks on Chávez, 18. *See also* Afro-Venezuelans; empowerment of historically disenfranchised groups; indigenous people; marginalization of historically disenfranchised groups
Race, Kane, 8
RCTV cable network, 72
Rebhun, Linda-Ann, 54
reciprocity of state-citizen relations, 156–57
red zone (*zona roja*), 26, 104
religion: biomedicine intertwined with, 31–35, 85–87, 164n1; Lionza, María, cult of (espiritismo), 32, 85, 86, 91, 164n2, 167nn19–20; Pentecostalism, 85; santería, 85, 90, 97, 167nn25–26; spiritual healing traditions, 85–87, 91, 167nn19–20,25–27,29. *See also* Catholicism; Hernández, José Gregorio (doctor-saint)
reproductive technologies (IVF), 8, 160n10
revolution: bias and skepticism about, 155; definition of, 154, 172n13; inevitable incompleteness of, 142; lack of ethnographies of, 154–55, 172n14; love as basis of, 59–60; pleasure and fun as important guiding ethics for, 156
right-wing opposition to Chávez-era government: overview, 17–18; attempts to remove Chávez from office (legal and extralegal), 18; class and, 149–50; community health workers harassed by members of, 115–16; and displeasure with empowerment of historically disenfranchised groups, 12; as "escuálidos" (squalid ones), 18, 51; government health care accessed by members of, 51; historically marginalized majority as rejecting, 148, 149–50, 172n6; participant narratives countering, 40–41, 164n8; and post-Chávez government, 148, 149–50, 151; and private health care, preference for, 40–41; racist attacks on Chávez, 18; universal public health care as accepted by, 21; violent

attacks on Barrio Adentro clinics and hospitals, 21, 151
Roberts, Elizabeth, 67, 160n10

Samet, Robert, 29
Santa Teresa (residential district): central plaza of, 25, 26, 113, 116, 118, 120, 127, 170n2; as field site, 24–27, 25–26, 127; and health care prior to Barrio Adentro, 27, 45; historical city center in, 128; inseguridad and, 26–27, 127, 138, 170n2; socioeconomic standing of neighborhood, 25–26. *See also* methodology
santería, 85, 90, 97, 167nn25–26
Schiller, Naomi, 29
Seventh Day Adventism, 85
Shah, Alpa, 155
Smilde, David, 163n83
Smith-Oka, Vania, 159n5
social inequalities: community-based medicine as challenge to, 44–46; neoliberal austerity measures and increases in, 16. *See also aprovechando* (making the most of government services); empowerment of historically disenfranchised groups; marginalization of historically disenfranchised groups; *participación popular* (popular participation)
socialist governments: and government support for popular/traditional medicine, 95; medical practices of, as reinforcing marginalization of historically disenfranchised groups, 71, 97. *See also* Chávez-era government; Cuba; empowerment of historically disenfranchised groups; national belonging; revolution
social justice: Chávez and emphasis on, 5–6, 18–19; Negra Hipólita mission for, 130; "social missions" and, 19. *See also* empowerment of historically disenfranchised groups
Social Security Administration (IVSS), and pre-Chávez health care, 14
soup kitchens (*casas de alimentación*), 23, 124, 136
Soviet Union (USSR), 71
Spain, Grandparents Clubs in, 169n6